DRY NEEDLING FOR
MANUAL THERAPISTS

of related interest

The Active Points Test
A Clinical Test for Identifying and Selecting Effective
Points for Acupuncture and Related Therapies
Stefano Marcelli
ISBN 978 1 84819 233 1
eISBN 978 0 85701 207 4

DRY NEEDLING FOR
MANUAL THERAPISTS

*Points, Techniques and Treatments,
Including Electroacupuncture and
Advanced Tendon Techniques*

Giles Gyer, Jimmy Michael and Ben Tolson

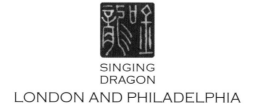

SINGING
DRAGON
LONDON AND PHILADELPHIA

Medical images provided by Alila Medical Images.
Photos taken by Frances Tolson (www.evokepictures.co.uk).

First published in 2016
by Singing Dragon
an imprint of Jessica Kingsley Publishers
73 Collier Street
London N1 9BE, UK
and
400 Market Street, Suite 400
Philadelphia, PA 19106, USA

www.singingdragon.com

Library of Congress Cataloging in Publication Data
A CIP catalog record for this book is available from the Library of Congress

British Library Cataloguing in Publication Data
A CIP catalogue record for this book is available from the British Library

ISBN 978 1 84819 255 3
eISBN 978 0 85701 202 9

Printed and bound in China

Contents

Part I

BACKGROUND

Chapter 1

Introduction

This book is primarily for health professionals who are treating musculoskeletal (MSK) conditions and who wish to incorporate acupuncture into their practice. We acknowledge that acupuncture can treat conditions other than MSK, but that is beyond the scope of the book.

Physical therapists see many MSK problems in clinic, which makes them ideal candidates to incorporate acupuncture into their practice. Musculoskeletal problems of various types are often the most common reasons for patients to seek care from acupuncturists, representing one third to one half of all visits (Sherman *et al.* 2005). In one study of Chinese patients (Mao *et al.* 2007), patients presented with pain-related musculoskeletal complaints such as back and neck pain (53%), arthritis (41%), neurological complaints such as post-stroke rehabilitation and facial paralysis (23%), and weight loss (10%). In the United Kingdom acupuncture is used in 84 per cent of chronic pain clinics (Woollam and Jackson 1998).

Acupuncture has become more accepted by Western medicine over the last 30 years and has seen an exponential growth in its practice worldwide (Guerreiro da Silva 2013). As the practice of acupuncture has grown, so too has the evidence base. The advantages of using acupuncture are well documented and include an immediate reduction in local, referred and widespread pain, restoration of range of motion and muscle activation patterns, and a normalization of the immediate chemical environment of active myofascial trigger points (Dommerholt 2011). As well as these well-documented effects, acupuncture can have simultaneous widespread effects at multiple sites.

Acupuncture as part of manual therapy is rarely a stand-alone procedure and should be part of a broader physical therapy approach. Other approaches, including soft tissue mobilization, manipulation, therapeutic exercise and functional retraining, should be used in combination with acupuncture. For example, after deactivation of myofascial trigger points, patients should be educated in appropriate self-care techniques which may include specific stretches of the involved muscles and self-massage techniques (American Physical Therapy Association 2013).

As the appetite for acupuncture has grown, there now exist varying standards of training. The requirements for acupuncture training have yet to be provided and vary considerably in practice. Broadly speaking there are two main training routes for acupuncture: courses for lay persons and courses for medically qualified practitioners.

Those courses which are mainly for lay persons are generally very comprehensive and will include a mixture of standard Western anatomy and pathology with a large percentage of traditional Chinese medicine (TCM). TCM theory is extremely complex, takes a long time to learn and includes pulse and tongue diagnosis amongst other techniques.

The courses attended by medically qualified practitioners are usually much shorter. This is because, in the case of doctors and allied health professionals, their knowledge of diagnosis, pathology, anatomy, physiology, microbiology and other treatment techniques that can be used at the same time as acupuncture can be taken for granted.

White (2009, p.33) defines dry needling (also know as Western medical acupuncture) as a 'therapeutic modality involving the insertion of fine needles; it is an adaptation of Chinese acupuncture using current knowledge of anatomy, physiology and pathology, and the principles of evidence-based medicine. Although Western medical acupuncture has evolved from Chinese acupuncture, its practitioners no longer adhere to concepts such as yin/yang and circulation of qi, and regard acupuncture as part of conventional medicine rather than a complete "alternative medical system".' For convenience, however, the term acupuncture will be used throughout this book.

Hong (2013, p.593) describes acupuncture as covering 'a diverse academic field that spans from ancient medical history to the most advanced contemporary neurophysiology'. He continues: 'Acupuncture as a treatment for pain encompasses much more than simply needling: it involves a complex interaction and context that may include empathy, touch, intention, attention, expectation and conditioning.'

The term 'dry needling' is often used to differentiate this technique from myofascial trigger point injections. Myofascial trigger point injections are performed with a variety of injectables, such as: procaine, lidocaine and other local anaesthetics; isotonic saline solutions; non-steroidal anti-inflammatories;

corticosteroids; bee venom; botulinum toxin; and serotonin antagonists (Dommerholt, del Moral and Gröbli 2006).

Many acupuncturists see the use of so-called dry needling/Western medical acupuncture as an infringement of the rights of traditional acupuncture practitioners. It is the position of some organizations that any intervention utilizing dry needling beyond trigger point dry needling is the practice of acupuncture, regardless of the language utilized in describing the technique. Acupuncturists will argue that by using acupuncture in their practice practitioners may inadvertently be affecting the whole organism without realizing it.

Whether acupuncture falls within the confines of a single discipline or should be incorporated into physical therapy remains a question to be answered by individuals and the respective organizations or governing bodies. Currently in some parts of the world this has resulted in a turf war where legislation has been passed banning the use of acupuncture within manual or physical therapy.

At its heart, Western medical acupuncture has a scientific rationale. Acupuncture training programmes must provide students with sufficient knowledge to communicate the science and theories underlying acupuncture in conventional medical language.

Resistance to implementation of broad integrative clinical training has encouraged other professions such as medicine, chiropractic and physical therapy to include acupuncture in their scope of practice, redefined as percutaneous electrical nerve stimulation, transcutaneous electrical nerve stimulation and dry needling (Dommerholt 2011), which explain the modality in conventional medical language (Stumpf, Kendall and Hardy 2010).

One current argument against acupuncture being used within modern healthcare settings in the West is that acupuncture mechanisms (how it works) cannot depend on a philosophical or political debate that transcends clinical practice (Stumpf *et al.* 2010). Only through a universal way to describe how acupuncture works, along with safe working practices and treatment strategies, will a continued adoption of acupuncture theory and understanding be promoted.

Stumpf *et al.* (2010) argue that the greatest barriers to integration, however, originate with acupuncture training programmes based on European metaphysical ideas (Kendall 2008) which therefore do not ensure that graduates have a sufficient understanding of quality biomedical knowledge and mainstream medicine, including primary care, or are able to evaluate research competently (Hammerschlag 2006). Without adequate knowledge or exposure to mainstream medicine, graduates are unprepared to (a) function effectively in an integrative healthcare team, (b) provide competent primary care to patients, or (c) make appropriate referrals to physicians and other mainstream providers.

The focus should be on expanding acupuncture to populations that might not necessarily be able to access acupuncture through private practice. Just as spinal manipulation should not be exclusive to one profession, so should the practice of acupuncture. Our hope is that traditional acupuncturists will study the known Western medical theories of how acupuncture works and will give a flavour of the understanding of how traditional acupuncture works from an energetic perspective. Only by ensuring high educational standards for training physical therapists will acupuncture be practised safely, and this book is not intended to replace such training.

Only by integrating different modalities such as acupuncture into our practice will patients benefit fully. The practice of integrative medicine has emerged as a potential solution to solve complex problems seen in our patient population (Maizes, Rakel and Niemiec 2009).

Good medicine is based on good science. It is inquiry-driven and open to new paradigms. It is both practical and pragmatic. Although Western acupuncture has evolved from TCM, we are not dismissing the TCM approach to acupuncture. Western medicine is continually evolving and the explanations given are based on current evidence. As the evidence continues to grow, we may be able to explain more of the mechanisms of acupuncture. There is now much positive evidence to support the use of acupuncture, and this is outlined later in the book.

The techniques in the book are the ones the authors frequently use in clinical practice. Obviously this book is intended only as a supplement for acupuncture training. Perhaps the use of acupuncture should be patient-centred and not driven by professional disputes. It is our hope that by writing this book more health professionals will be able to use acupuncture in their practice and help the many patients who are suffering in pain.

References

American Physical Therapy Association (APTA) (2013) *Description of Dry Needling in Clinical Practice.* Alexandria, VA: APTA Public Policy, Practice, and Professional Affairs Unit. Available at www.apta.org/StateIssues/DryNeedling/ClinicalPracticeResourcePaper, accessed on 15 July 2015.

Dommerholt, J. (2011) 'Dry needling – peripheral and central considerations.' *Journal of Manual and Manipulative Therapies 19*, 4, 223–227.

Dommerholt, J., del Moral, O.M., and Gröbli, C. (2006) 'Trigger point dry needling.' *Journal of Manual & Manipulative Therapy 14*, 4, E70–E87.

Guerreiro da Silva, J.B. (2013) 'Integrative medicine, integrative acupuncture.' *European Journal of Integrative Medicine 5*, 83–86.

Hammerschlag, R. (2006) 'Evidence-based complementary and alternative medicine: back to basics.' *Journal of Alternative and Complementary Medicine 12*, 349–350.

Hong, H. (2013) *Acupuncture: Theories and Evidence.* Singapore: World Scientific Publishing.

Kendall, D.E. (2008) 'Energy – meridian misconceptions of Chinese medicine.' *Schweiz. Zschr. GanzheitsMedizin 20*, 2, 112–117.

Maizes, V., Rakel, D., and Niemiec, C.J.D. (2009) 'Integrative medicine and patient centred care.' *Explore (NY) 5*, 5, 277–289. Commissioned for the IOM Summit on Integrative Medicine and the Health of the Public.

Mao, J.J., Farrar, J.T., Armstrong, K., Donahue, A., Ngo, J., and Bowman, M.A. (2007) 'De qi: Chinese acupuncture patients' experiences and beliefs regarding acupuncture needling sensation – an exploratory survey.' *Acupunct. Med. 25*, 4, 158–165.

Sherman, K.J., Cherkin, D.C., Eisenberg, D.M., *et al.* (2005) 'The practice of acupuncture: who are the providers and what do they do?' *Annals of Family Medicine 3*, 151–158.

Stumpf, S.H., Kendall, D.E., and Hardy, M.L. (2010) 'Mainstreaming acupuncture: barriers and solutions.' *Journal of Evidence-Based Complementary & Alternative Medicine 15*, 1, 3–13.

White, A. (2009) 'Western medical acupuncture: a definition.' *Acupunct. Med. 27*, 33–35.

Woollam, C.H.M., and Jackson, A.O. (1998) 'Acupuncture in the management of chronic pain.' *Journal of Anaesthesia 53*, 593–595.

Chapter 2

A Short History of Acupuncture

It is important for the practitioner to have an understanding of the origins of acupuncture as it puts current practice into context. Also, it is useful to understand some of the principles and techniques in traditional Chinese medicine (TCM), as it is from these techniques that Western acupuncture has evolved. Some clinical trials and research papers may also use TCM methodology and traditional acupuncture points, so being able to understand and evaluate the treatment protocols and locations is of benefit when forming one's own clinical reasoning and opinions of such research. This chapter outlines some current thinking in TCM and how that might differ from a Western medical approach.

Before the discussion of the origins of acupuncture begins, it must be stated that acupuncture is just one part of an ancient medical system. Typically there are four main disciplines that form part of TCM:

- acupuncture

- herbal medicine

- Chinese massage/bodywork/physical therapy known as tui na (which means 'push and grasp')

- Chinese exercise such as martial arts, tai chi, qi gong and esoteric practices.

These disciplines are still in use in China and other parts of the Orient today and, when combined, provide a powerful tool for healing. Treatments draw from all aspects of Oriental medicine: acupuncture, bodywork, exercise, meditation and herbal medicine.

For example, in China, tui na is one of the most commonly used modalities in the practice of TCM. It includes techniques such as pushing (*tui*) and grasping (*na*) of soft tissue. Tui na is a manual therapy based on the principles of TCM aimed at restoring health and treating various clinical conditions, primarily MSK conditions. Tui na has developed and is now incorporated into other clinical disciplines, such as acupuncture, gynaecology and paediatrics. Tui na uses a variety of manual techniques guided by the theory of TCM. The philosophy of TCM strongly influences the attitude and approach of tui na practitioners towards healthcare (World Health Organization 2010).

The practice of herbal medicine is one that can be traced back to the third century AD where the classification of herbs had already begun. The classification continued and was documented in works such as *The Compendium of Materia Medica*, an impressive 52 volumes that described 1892 herbs. In clinical practice, traditional diagnosis may be followed by the prescription of complex and often individualized remedies. Although animal and mineral materials have been used, the primary source of remedies is botanical. Herbs are taken individually or as part of a prescription where a combination of herbs is used, typically between six and nine herbs per prescription. A herbalist's entire pharmacy may contain between 200 and 600 potential substances (Yuen *et al.* 2012).

The use of herbal remedies is widespread in China. Ergil, Kramer and Ng (2002, p.2) describe the extent of herbal medicine as follows: 'It was once customary for families to have a household repertoire of herbal formulae to treat medical problems and to address life changes (pregnancy, menopause, old age) and the seasons. Some families retain, and especially older patients may continue to follow, these practices.' Large pharmaceutical companies are currently investing and researching the active ingredients in many of the herbs used in TCM.

Lewith (1982) describes the first attempt at recording disease dating back to around 1500 BC during the Shang Dynasty. Tortoise shells with inscriptions were found, and it is thought that these were used for divination in the art of healing. As with much of TCM's history, the philosophical basis of many of these findings indicates that practitioners sought to seek harmony between the living and their dead ancestors, and the good and evil spirits that inhabited the earth.

Another huge milestone in the development of acupuncture is *The Yellow Emperor's Canon of Internal Medicine*. This is the first Chinese medical text to describe acupuncture and is in a question-and-answer format between the

Yellow Emperor and one of his ministers. The academic divergence of thoughts in this book sufficiently indicates that it is neither a work of a single individual, nor medical achievement of a certain period or a local region, but rather the summarization of experiences of many medical practitioners over a long time. This text dates possibly (as sources vary) to as early as the second century BC. Later texts evolved and included a description of the channels (acupuncture channels), functions of the acupuncture points, needling techniques, types of qi, description of diseases and location of acupuncture points.

Collectively these early but comprehensive texts are known as the Chinese medical classics and are the philosophical foundation for the practice of Chinese medicine. TCM practitioners continually refer back to these sources to inform current practice. These documents contain a comprehensive source of theoretical and clinical information (Neal 2013).

Main sources of knowledge and development

The roots of acupuncture and Chinese medicine developed over a long period of time, drawing upon a variety of sources. Wang Ju-Yi and Robertson (2008) and Denmei (2003) describe six main sources of knowledge and development of acupuncture.

1. Early massage

Every early civilization has some form of touch therapy and China is no exception. Massage therapy predates acupuncture and is still in use today. Massage therapy is called tui na in China, translated as *tui* (push) and *na* (grasp), giving an insight into how it works. It was previously called an mo: *an* (pressing) and *mo* (rubbing). Acupuncturists will often use tui na alongside acupuncture for more effective treatments, and when studying in China students have to learn both tui na and acupuncture, giving an indication of the close relationship of the two separate disciplines.

Through time this tui na grew into a cohesive body of knowledge and was used to treat a variety of conditions. The practice of tui na can focus on painful areas, acupuncture points and acupuncture channels. Today the range of conditions treated by tui na includes musculoskeletal conditions, gynaecology, paediatrics and rehabilitation, and the technique is widely used in hospitals throughout China. A good example of its use in the treatment of childhood diseases was first described in the book *The Massage of Lao Zi* by

Dr Sun Si Miao (AD 590–682). Infantile tui na was the treatment of choice during imperial times, especially integrated with gao mo (the application of external herbal preparations as ointments/tinctures/pastes).

One proposition is that pressing on certain points away from painful areas relieved pain/discomfort. For example, rubbing a point near the wrist relieved stomach ache. This led to practitioners searching for more points away from the area of pain that would relieve the main complaint. Over time more areas and points were found and used on a frequent basis to help a wide variety of conditions. Particular points were more effective for certain conditions and that knowledge was passed on to other practitioners and eventually was written down. This discovery was probably a major contributor to the development of acupuncture and was invaluable in the treatment of pain and disease.

As more practitioners used touch to search and identify points, other noticeable changes were found on the body they were working on. It was discovered that certain points and areas showed signs of disease before disease presented itself. This discovery aided the early practitioners in diagnosing disease before it had manifested and enabled them to use this information as a diagnostic aid.

It is unclear when the introduction of inserting needles into points on the body first started. Early stone needles were in use for bloodletting and perhaps these were used initially as primitive acupuncture needles. Eventually metal needles were used, made from bronze, gold or silver. Today the modern needles are made from surgical stainless steel.

Perhaps the early practitioners had too many points to massage at one time (they simply didn't have enough hands!), so tried inserting needles. Perhaps the points needed longer stimulation for better effects; or the better the practitioner became, the more patients and less time he had? Some of the acupuncture points are extremely small and are often found in between joint spaces, so maybe this required something finer than a thumb or finger. Also, using acupuncture needles is less labour-intensive than using thumbs or fingers. Other theories are that the needle was an extension of the thumb, enabling practitioners to enter the channels more deeply in order to contact, engage and manipulate qi for particular therapeutic effects such as cooling, draining and dispersing.

Denmei (2003) suggests that acupuncture needles developed from the needles used in sewing and were adapted for use for acupuncture. Seamstresses would sew for long hours and develop shoulder and neck pain. Perhaps the pain got so bad one day that a needle was inserted into the tight neck and shoulders and relieved the pain. Once needles were used, practitioners discovered just how effective needling was and the practice grew from there, which echoes the situation today.

2. Historical autopsy

There are many early accounts of physicians examining and listing the location, size and weight of organs. These examinations formed the basis of anatomical drawings and locations of major organs. They named the organs and described their functions. In fact, more than 2000 years ago, they knew that the heart is the organ that pumps blood through the body. This was not discovered in Western medicine until the early sixteenth century.

The anatomical location of the major organs played an important part in the development of medical knowledge. Historically, though, China was isolated from the medical developments in Europe, so many of the scientific ideas remained unchallenged. The Chinese formulated ideas that stated that health consisted of the interaction of qi, blood and body fluids. Some of these ideas will be expanded on later.

3. Surgery

Early surgery was performed when no other option was available, and this again informed the medical profession. Physicians would attend these operations and observe what took place. China has a long history of brutal wars, and the physicians who treated the wounded and dying would draw upon their experience to formulate medical ideas.

Chinese surgeons, given the unavailability of anaesthetics, wisely restricted their procedures to the surface of the body where operations could be performed quickly with a minimum of discomfort without the necessity for muscular relaxation (Zaroff 1999). Neal (2013), from his studies of the *Nei Jing*, suggests that acupuncture was the primary intervention for emergency conditions similar to those for which surgery is performed today.

Kan-Wen Ma (2000) gives one such example when, in the year 1034, the Emperor was sick and imperial doctors were having no success in treating him, so an acupuncturist called Xu Xi was recommended and summoned. After examining the Emperor, he announced that he could cure him if he were allowed to insert needles between the external membranes below the

Emperor's heart. The court physicians deemed the procedure extremely dangerous and therefore tested the method first on their own bodies. The procedure was declared safe and Xu Xi was allowed to treat the Emperor. The treatment was successful, and as a result Xu Xi was appointed medical officer of the Imperial Medical Institute.

4. Qi gong, tai chi and martial arts

Qi gong, literally energy (*qi*) skill (*gong*), is an ancient Chinese healing art involving meditation, controlled breathing and movement exercises designed to improve physical and mental wellbeing and prevent disease. The aims of such exercises are to nourish, cultivate, balance and increase awareness of qi (pronounced 'chee'), our life force. Qi gong therapy is an important branch of traditional Chinese medicine, which has a history of thousands of years and is still used today to prevent diseases and treat illness around the world.

For example, qi gong exercises are often prescribed to patients as part of their treatment plan. Just as a physiotherapist would give patients stretches and exercises, so too a qi gong doctor would prescribe qi gong exercises. Meditation also might be prescribed to patients. Qi gong and other forms of Chinese exercises are performed daily in the parks in China and are a common sight.

Qi gong is often translated as 'energy work' and can be considered to be both body and mind medicine. Undoubtedly, practitioners of this art helped discover the acupuncture channels and points by the regular practice of qi gong. Practitioners of qi gong through regular practice are able to feel qi in their body. The more experience one has with qi gong, the more one feels the flow of energy in the body through the different acupuncture channels. These sensations, felt by practitioners over thousands of years, were documented and formed part of the knowledge that led to the development of acupuncture and TCM theory.

Throughout Chinese history, numerous acupuncturists have been qi gong experts, and the practice of qi gong has helped their skill level. Qi gong shares many of the same theoretical foundations as acupuncture.

Qi gong's popularity in China cannot be underestimated. As Deadman (2014, p.10) declares: 'At the height of its popularity in China in the 1980s, it is estimated that one hundred million people were practising qigong in parks and public spaces. Crowds flocked to hear great masters speak and to be healed simply by being in their presence or hearing their words. Prime-time television showed miraculous acts being performed by the power of qi while China's top scientists and politicians were caught up in an extraordinary vision of qigong releasing the supernormal powers latent in human beings.'

As a healing modality, the practice of qi gong in TCM matches that of acupuncture and tui na. Acupuncture and tui na – especially acupuncture – cannot be separated from an understanding of the channels (channels and qi), and ancient people considered the discovery of the channels directly related to qi gong.

Acupuncture points have also been used in martial arts. A style of martial arts known as dim mak makes extensive use of striking certain acupuncture points with devastating effects. The acupuncture points are over major nerves and blood vessels and the most vulnerable parts of the neck and skull, so striking them can cause considerable pain. Different results are possible depending on which point or combination of points are hit and how they are hit, much like acupuncture but with an entirely different intent. There is an entire branch of Chinese medicine devoted to repairing beaten-up martial artists, called dit dar, which is itself another great story of Chinese medicine. Briefly, dit dar could be considered as a combination of skills including bone setting, a manipulation similar to chiropractic and osteopathy, but which also uses massage, qi gong and external herbs to facilitate healing.

5. Clinical and empirical experience

If a treatment worked, then usually it was written down, repeated and further refined. If a treatment did not work, then it was abandoned and fell out of use. Acupuncture points are undoubtedly the end-product of millions of detailed observations. As they were developed, so each of them was given a name and Chinese character, depending on its therapeutic properties. Particular acupuncture points were noted relating to which conditions they were useful at treating, and this recording of knowledge continues to this day. In clinical practice, a set of acupuncture points are selected for treatment in order to produce a specific effect in the body.

6. Philosophy

As with any system of medicine, acupuncture was influenced by the ideas of the time. Influential philosophical ideas stemmed from Buddhism, Daoism and Confucianism along with the observation of the seasons and nature. All these aspects had their part to play in informing ideas about the developments of disease from birth to death.

The Chinese considered the human body to be a microcosm of the universe and world. Part of this idea is the concept of yin and yang. Yin and yang are thought to be the essential components of all living things. For example, dualities such as light and dark, fire and water and male and female are thought of as physical manifestations of the duality of yin and yang. The taijitu symbol is an example of this concept. This Chinese symbol represents yin and yang existing in harmony and shows how they give rise to each other as they interrelate with one another.

Some basic principles of TCM

In TCM the individual structures of the body are also assigned to be either yin or yang in nature. The organs in TCM are known as the zang fu. The zang organs are the 'solid' organs and are yin in nature, and the fu organs are the 'hollow' organs and are yang in nature.

The stomach, small intestine, large intestine, bladder and gallbladder are all yang. The yin organs are considered to be the heart, lungs, kidneys, spleen and liver. The yin and yang aspects of the body counterbalance each other. A deficit of one naturally leads to a surfeit of the other, while a surfeit of one will weaken the other. In both cases, yin and yang no longer counterbalance each other, and disease arises as a result. Nothing is ever completely yin or yang, but a combination of the two. These two principles are always interacting, opposing and influencing each other. The goal of Chinese medicine is not to eliminate either yin or yang, but to allow the two to balance each other and for the energies' influences to exist harmoniously together. Ultimately, every modality within TCM is aimed at regulating yin and yang, to balance yin and yang.

In addition to the zang fu there are the extraordinary fu organs which are characterized by hollowness, similar to the six fu organs in morphology, and storage of essence, similar to the five zang organs in function. This group of tissues and organs are the brain, the marrow, the bones, the vessels, the gallbladder and the uterus.

Acupuncture points were subsequently grouped into a system of channels which run over the body, conducting the flow of vital energy through the body. The acupuncture points on a channel are said to influence the flow of vital energy through the channel, thereby influencing disease processes within the body. As a further representation of the human body in the natural world, the current of energy and fluids of the body are sometimes referred to as channels, seas, rivers and reservoirs. There are 12 main primary acupuncture channels, and each channel is considered to be connected to an organ; for example, there is the large intestine channel, and so on.

In addition to the 12 main primary channels there are also eight extra channels. This is because they have independent points – points that are not on any of the 12 regular channels. There are also so-called extra points that are not located on the 12 main channels. Xie (2008) gives the analogy that 'qi-passage' is in fact the essence of the channel-collateral system in the human body (more on this later in the book). He goes on to state (p.4) that 'the so-called "Jing" of the fourteen channels is referred to the tissue structure of the longitudinal fascia space; the so-called "Luo" of the fifteen collaterals is referred to the tissue structure of the transversal fascia space, and the "Mai" of channels and collaterals is referred to tissue liquid-qi of both longitudinal and transversal fascia space'. An in-depth discussion of fascia and the acupuncture channel systems is presented in later chapters.

For further clarification, the Chinese named each acupuncture point and also numbered each acupuncture point along the course of the channel assigned to each organ. For example, the heart channel has nine acupuncture points running from the armpit down the inner surface of the arm to the tip of the little finger, whereas the bladder channel has a total of 67 points.

Qi

Qi is the word which encompasses the meaning of all vital activities and substances in the human body. It is the 'life force' of all living things as well as representative of all energy within the universe. It is beyond a simple definition, but is the key to understanding Eastern philosophy and the unique holistic approach when assessing health in humans.

According to TCM, our health and wellbeing is dependent on the body's vital energy, our qi, moving in a smooth and balanced way through a series of channels beneath the skin. The energy of a person's body is distributed along 12 main acupuncture channels which run up and down the body, connecting and linking the different organs and parts of the body with one another, creating a living interconnecting network that can be easily accessed. The acupuncturist taps into the network of channels and guides the body to begin its own healing process.

During a treatment a fine, single-use, sterile stainless steel needle is inserted just below the surface of the skin to stimulate acupuncture points lying along the acupuncture channels which run throughout the body to activate or unblock the flow of energy, restoring balance and triggering the body's natural healing response. Health is seen as a state of physical, mental and social wellbeing accompanied by freedom from illness or pain.

In TCM theory, every organ has its own qi. For example, when the heart becomes weak, known as weak heart qi, a person can experience palpitations. When someone has weak lung qi they have problems breathing or may be asthmatic. Each organ will have signs and symptoms when malfunctioning, which the practitioner will search for whilst looking for disharmony. Thus, traditional Chinese models of health and restoration are concerned with the function of the organs. By assessing each organ function through questioning and diagnosis, this leads the practitioner to a 'pattern of disharmony' that affects one or more organs. Treatment is then aimed at restoring the harmony by selecting a point on the appropriate acupuncture channel and stimulating that point. An over-simplistic example would be needling an acupuncture point such as Heart 7, shen men, which is on the heart channel and is said to regulate the heart.

Western observers often thought that the acupuncture channels were in fact blood vessels and qi was blood. Western practitioners have dismissed much of TCM theory because of lack of evidence of these channels and no definable way of measuring this so-called energy. In addition, the diagnostic methods used often seemed chaotic to the Western mind and based on unfamiliar concepts which were extremely subjective, making them unreliable tools.

Pulse diagnosis

A common tool amongst TCM practitioners is the examination of the radial pulse on both wrists. Three fingers are placed on the radial pulse and superficial and deep pressure applied to all three positions. Different positions and depths correspond to different organs.

The practitioner detects the rate, width, amplitude and length of each pulse position, which then gives them information about the state of balance of the body as a whole and the state of individual organs. There are, generally speaking, 29 different pulse qualities that can be assigned to each pulse position. Pulse diagnosis takes time to master, but practitioners would not have spent this considerable time unless they had found it to be a useful diagnostic tool.

Tongue diagnosis

Another key diagnostic tool in TCM is tongue diagnosis. The tongue has many relationships and connections in the body, and is considered to be a reflection of the internal organs with different areas of the tongue representing different organs. Tongue diagnosis gives visual indicators of a person's overall health. When examining the tongue, the practitioner looks at the colour of the tongue body, its size and shape, the colour and thickness of its coating, movement such as quivering, and moistness or dryness of the tongue body. By itself tongue diagnosis is not a stand-alone diagnostic tool, but the information from it is taken as part of an overall pattern.

In TCM, health implies that the body system is in a state of dynamic equilibrium, not only between the various parts of the body but also between the body and environmental conditions. The final diagnosis is based on the information gathered from all the above-mentioned diagnostic methods. These methods are not used in isolation, but as parts of a system. From patient questioning and examination, the information gathered is matched to a corresponding TCM pattern. Pattern identification is the process used in TCM that enables a practitioner to determine the significance of symptoms and to create a coherent picture of a client's state of ill/wellbeing. TCM differentiates biomedical diseases into patterns. Each pattern comprises symptoms/signs that have their own unique treatment protocol. This is the TCM clinical reasoning model and further breaks down patterns into organ dysfunctions, channel disorders or local injury. This system gives TCM a holistic approach towards the sick individual, and disturbances are treated at the physical, emotional, mental, spiritual and environmental levels simultaneously.

Moxibustion

Acupuncture (zhen jiu) means the act of needling and moxibustion. The *Huang Di Nei Jing* states: 'If the disease cannot be treated successfully with acupuncture, it will be treated with moxibustion.' In other words the two cannot be separated. Moxibustion has received far less attention in the West, and much of the knowledge and experience has been left to one side or ignored.

Moxibustion is the method of burning the herb mugwort on, around or above acupuncture points for therapeutic purposes. The leaves of the mugwort are dried and ground to the right consistency so that it can bind well together. Moxa is typically rolled into balls for use for burning on acupuncture points, shaped into cones to put on top of acupuncture needles, or it can be bought in prepackaged tiny or long rolls known as moxa sticks to warm large areas of the body. The advantage of moxa over other types of herb or plant is that it holds together well, burns evenly, is inexpensive and is widely available. Interestingly the practice of moxibustion was widespread in ancient China due to its relative safety and ease of practice compared with acupuncture, which would have carried a certain amount of risk (Wang Xue Tai 1984).

One possible explanation for moxa to be chosen is that certain religious rites, and divination for healing purposes, led to the direct use of burning by incense or tree branches on the body itself for healing. In fact, mugwort was also used for divination, and it is perhaps as a result of this that mugwort was chosen as the best plant for moxibustion (Maciocia 1982).

Development of acupuncture needles

The majority of people prefer not to be punctured with needles, and associate needling with pain and injury. Many plants and animals have evolved thorns or quills as powerful weapons for protection or attack, so this represents a barrier to many people even considering having acupuncture and raises the question as to how acupuncture came and stayed in use throughout history (Xinghua 2008).

A good case highlighting fear of needles occurred in 1945, when Japan was occupied by the Allied Forces. The Japanese government was ordered to ban acupuncture and moxibustion as a barbarous and unscientific therapy. This was due to the fact that some Japanese soldiers used acupuncture or moxibustion on Allied Forces prisoners of war (POWs), with good intentions because of the medical supply shortage, but the POWs took it as a form of torture, and some of those Japanese soldiers were subsequently indicted as war criminals.

Other stories surrounding the birth of acupuncture include tales of soldiers who were cured of an illness/disease after being shot with an arrow. Other accounts suggest that the practice of bloodletting had a part to play. Bloodletting is the practice of withdrawal of blood to cure disease and illness. The tools used for bloodletting may have been available to practitioners to experiment with.

The first needles are widely considered to have been made of stone, examples of which have been found in ancient tombs excavated in Inner Mongolia and Hunan Province. Maciocia (1982) describes three kinds of stone needles with varying degrees of sharpness. The sharpest were probably used to make incisions to let out pus, while the blunt ones were probably used for some kind of skin-scraping.

After stone, needles were made principally of bone and bamboo. During the Bronze Age the introduction of bronze needles began, and later other metals were used, including silver and gold from around 500 BC. Other evidence indicates that jade was also used, and by 200 BC steel was available (Maciocia 1982). The manufacture of acupuncture needles today is thankfully very sophisticated and has evolved with patient comfort in mind. The needles are often made of high-grade steel and the tips are highly polished to provide a very smooth needle insertion.

Brief overview of acupuncture development in modern China

It must be remembered that acupuncture has not always enjoyed the popularity it has today. Throughout China's history it has suffered periods of decline. Often it symbolized old, backward ways of thinking in direct opposition to those people who wanted to modernize China. One such example was in 1929 when the Ministry of Health limited the advertising of TCM and prohibited the establishment of any teaching of TCM.

In 1928 the Communist Party of China was formed, under the leadership of Chairman Mao. A long guerrilla war ensued and the Communist Party finally took power in 1949. The Communists had little or no medical services in the 'liberated areas' and actively encouraged the use of traditional Chinese remedies to keep their troops on the move. These remedies were cheap, acceptable to the Chinese peasants, and utilized the skills already available in the countryside. There were around 12,000 Western-trained doctors – a staggering one doctor for every 26,000 people in China. Traditional doctors such as acupuncturists, herbalists and tui na practitioners were estimated to be around 400,000 in number.

China needed to establish a cost-effective care system that could be duplicated and provide health for all of its citizens. Essentially China could not afford to train a large number of doctors in Western medicine; however, it could easily afford to train large numbers of people in traditional medicine and thereby promote traditional methods of Chinese medicine and integrate them into mainstream medicine. There were many contradictory theories and practices in China at that time, and schools which practised traditional medicine in China were standardized and systematized similar to a Western-style university. During this period an attempt was made to unify the various family, regional and theoretical schools of acupuncture throughout China – a seemingly impossible task. The new teaching model was in direct contrast to the previous student–master apprenticeship. In order to teach large numbers of people, the medicine of the time had to be standardized.

During the early 1950s many hospitals opened clinics to provide, teach and investigate the traditional methods. This renaissance of acupuncture, combined with a sophisticated scientific approach, has allowed the development of many new methods of acupuncture. This is reflected in some hospitals in China where a variety of disciplines are all working in unison under one roof, including Western doctors, acupuncturists, herbalists, radiologists and so on.

The Great Cultural Revolution was a ten-year political campaign led by Chairman Mao from 1966 to 1976 – a social experiment aimed at rekindling revolutionary fervour and purifying the party. Mao shut down the nation's schools, calling for a massive youth mobilization to take current party leaders to task for their embrace of bourgeois values and lack of revolutionary spirit. One of Mao's beliefs was that the progress China had made since 1949 had led to a privileged class developing, including engineers, scientists, managers and teachers.

As part of this great purge many surgeons and Western medicine doctors were thought to be too elitist and therefore were persecuted. TCM was also hailed as a national treasure and a great symbol for China. It must be remembered that, in 1942, Mao had ordered the government to banish all superstitious and shamanic beliefs, so his new appraisal and approval of TCM was a popular political move. TCM practitioners were not exempt from persecution, and many senior key figures were executed or expelled. A further part of healthcare reform, as emphasized in Mao's speech given in Beijing on 26 June 1965, was to abolish all entrance exams, and the training provided to TCM entrants was minimal. This led to the so-called 'barefoot doctors' who were sent out with very little training to address the medical needs of the vast majority of the Chinese who lived in the countryside.

The persecution of the medical establishment and the new medical reforms meant that medical learning was now open to the under-privileged classes such as peasants and general workers. This resulted in acupuncture having to replace Western medicine in many areas, and acupuncturists had the opportunity of gaining experience in many new areas. As part of this experimentation many new therapies emerged, propelled by the fear that they would face the same fate as their predecessors if they failed. Estimates vary, but roughly 1.5 million people were killed during the Cultural Revolution, and millions of others suffered imprisonment, seizure of property, torture or general humiliation, the aftermath of which still affects China's politics today.

Maciocia (1982) reports that during the Cultural Revolution the new methods of acupuncture included:

- ear acupuncture

- scalp acupuncture

- cat-gut surgery

- needle-embedding therapy

- point-injection therapy

- long needle therapy

- acupuncture analgesia

- electrical acupuncture.

Many of these new methods were influenced by Western medicine. For example, scalp acupuncture is a technique that has developed from the neuro-anatomy of the central nervous system. When the brain is damaged, such as due to a stroke, the scalp is stimulated superficially over the area of damaged brain (Lewith 1982).

To present TCM as a cohesive whole would be misleading, because as a result of standardization many lineages and styles of acupuncture were excluded when TCM schools and institutions were founded. What TCM does represent is a starting block for the practitioner to begin and to explore other styles of acupuncture later on. It is important to note that there is more than one style of acupuncture in existence and more than one way of practising acupuncture within TCM. Entirely different acupuncture modalities have developed and evolved without being incorporated into TCM. The acupuncture that has been exported/imported to the West may represent just a small sample of acupuncture theory and practice. However, what was taught was clinically verified, and many of the superstitious theories were excluded from modern textbooks.

Part of this unification of methodology included applying the methodology that was used in the practice of herbal medicine to acupuncture. Many of the practitioners involved in the unification of ideas were herbalists – therefore, they simply applied the diagnostic principles that were in use for the prescription of herbs to acupuncture. Thus a diagnosis would involve first a pattern discrimination, based upon looking, listening, asking and pulse/palpation. This would lead to treatment principles and to a treatment plan, with the treatment plan including the use of basic points. Acupuncture points were also given theoretical functions again so as to fit the formulaic approach. This approach is often criticized for using a repertoire of only the most basic points. Another criticism of the standardization of acupuncture is that it resulted in the loss of palpatory techniques central to the diagnosis in acupuncture. For example, the technique of channel palpation involves palpating the pathways of the 12 main channels to look for diagnostic tissue changes. Vital tools such as this can help refine and focus both the diagnosis and treatment but are often not taught in modern acupuncture schools and are absent in many acupuncture clinics, leading to acupuncture's ineffectiveness.

As China develops, it is keen to train more Western doctors; the number of physicians trained in Western medicine has soared. Current estimates are that China has 2.3 million doctors, 90 per cent of whom are trained in Western medicine (Sussmutt-Dyckorhoff and Wang 2010).

The Chinese government still to this day promotes the development of a modern TCM industry, as well as the integration of TCM into the national healthcare system and the integrated training of healthcare practitioners. This is reflected in both training and the building and infrastructure of modern hospitals. TCM is often integrated within the major hospitals engaged with both the specialization and integration of Western medicine. TCM within hospitals may range (depending on size) from having busy inpatient and outpatient wards for musculoskeletal problems, to herbal dispensaries and qi gong wards where exercises are prescribed. TCM is also included in the syllabus of most medical universities.

Acupuncture in Japan

Throughout history there has been an exchange of knowledge between China and Japan, and Chinese ideas and medicines were a vital part of this knowledge exchange. Traditional Japanese medicine has been used for 1500 years and includes herbal medicine, acupuncture, moxibustion and acupressure. One of the earliest-known introductions was in AD 552 when the Chinese Emperor presented an acupuncture book to the Japanese Emperor. Later, in AD 562, a Chinese man, Zhi Cong, brought an acupuncture book, *Illustrations of Channels and Points*, and other medical works to Japan (Kan-Wen Ma 2000).

Many schools of acupuncture were set up in Japan, and students were sent to China or Korea to bring back knowledge of acupuncture.

In 1635 the Edo government closed its borders with neighbouring countries, beginning a period of isolation that lasted for around 200 years. As a result an acupuncture developed within Japan that was free from outside influences, and over time the Japanese transformed the ideas, skills and medicines into modalities that were uniquely Japanese. There are a few key developments and stories that must be taken into account to appreciate how Japanese acupuncture has developed (Kobayashi, Uefuji and Yasumo 2010).

Japanese acupuncture significantly differs from other styles in its delicacy, preferring shallower needling and less stimulation than TCM in China. One of the most interesting facts about the development of Japanese acupuncture is that for the last 350 years some of the leading figures in its development have been blind. Estimates vary, but around 30 per cent of acupuncturists in Japan are blind. The concept of blind practitioners using needles may initially seem somewhat strange to us in the West; however, it is well known that people who lose one sense have a greater sensitivity within another area. The blind develop an extra capacity in the senses of hearing and touch.

In 1680 the first school to teach acupuncture and massage to the blind was established. This was the world's first organized vocational school for the physically handicapped, an innovation in itself. From that time, many acupuncture schools for the blind were built all over the country. In Japan, the practice of acupuncture utilizes the enhanced tactile skill of the blind and provides a profession where they may naturally excel (it must be stressed that not all blind people in Japan want to be acupuncturists and some feel frustrated by their limited job options). A large group of blind practitioners continue to influence both the practice and theory of acupuncture and massage in modern-day Japan; moreover, it is still believed that acupuncture and massage are occupations for the blind.

For example, Kodo Fukushima founded the Toyohari association in 1959 after losing his sight during the war and later qualified as an acupuncturist. The Toyohari association was developed primarily for blind acupuncturists. It emphasizes practical hands-on skills as opposed to large amounts of theory, placing an emphasis on abdominal palpation. Members meet regularly in small groups to practise, exchange ideas and present papers to each other as part of their ongoing training (Fixler and Kivity 1988).

A blind acupuncturist, Waichi Sugiyama, created a method for inserting a needle using a tube. In this technique a needle is put into a thin tube before inserting it in the body. This technique is now commonplace within acupuncture. As a result of this innovative technique, practitioners could now insert the needle with less pain, and consequently the use of thinner needles became common in Japan. This may not seem such an innovation until you consider that, until that time, the main needle insertion technique was a method where the needle is inserted directly into the body and tapped with a hammer. Evolving from thinner needles, the Japanese did not emphasize obtaining strong deqi during treatment. Instead they believed that the channel system responds to more gentle, light stimuli.

Acupuncture and massage schools were set up for the blind in Japan where traditional skills were taught. A refined sense of palpation is one of the defining features of Japanese acupuncture. Palpation is an important diagnostic tool: it dictates which points are chosen for treatment, rather than choosing according to disease or theory. This again developed because a blind practitioner has to rely on his sense of touch as opposed to any grand theory about which points may or may not work. Also, point location is not always at the exact location prescribed in traditional anatomical charts. Points are found again by palpation. The idea that a point would be treated without palpation first is alien to many Japanese practitioners.

Another diagnostic significance between the two styles is the use of abdominal palpation. In China the palpation of the pulses is used, which may be in part due to being culturally more acceptable and less intimate or invasive than abdominal or body palpation. In contrast, Japanese acupuncturists use the abdomen, known as the hara, as part of diagnosis to determine the health or otherwise of the patient – particularly, but not exclusively, the state of the abdominal organs or tissues and the related energy fields (Birch and Massutato 1993). This is partly due to the practical influence blind acupuncturists have exerted on Japanese acupuncture having a more hands-on approach.

Practitioners of Japanese acupuncture also confirm that the needle technique causes an immediate and noticeable change, usually by noticing changes in the pulse, to which they pay a great deal of attention, or by confirmation of changes in abdominal reflex areas. Feedback from the patient is critical to guiding the treatment and confirms that an energetic change has taken place.

During the nineteenth century in Japan, the introduction of Western medicine led to the political leaders of the time, believing it to be superior to acupuncture, seeking acupuncture's demise. Despite this, acupuncture continued to be practised in Japan as Western medicine was often expensive and only available in the major cities, whereas acupuncture and traditional medicine was accessible and easily accessed. Acupuncture was also exported to Korea and Vietnam through trade routes, scholars and practitioners.

The spread of acupuncture to the West

It was through contact and trade with Japan that Dutch medical practitioners observed the use of acupuncture and moxibustion. One such Dutch physician was William Ten Rhijne, who observed the use of acupuncture at Nagasaki Bay, where he was stationed for two years. Ten Rhijne was one of the travelling doctors of the Dutch East India Company and witnessed how acupuncture was practised and was impressed by its therapeutic effects and techniques. Ten Rhijne's 1683 essay *De Acupuntura* was the first substantial work to introduce acupuncture to a wider Western audience. It focused on practical acupuncture and moxibustion techniques rather than the theory behind them.

Also during the seventeenth century, Jesuit missionaries had travelled to China and had observed the practice of acupuncture. The Jesuit missionaries understood the language, and as a result their documentation of acupuncture included not just the practice of acupuncture but also included pulse diagnosis. They understood that acupuncture was based on the circulation of qi and were even able to translate Chinese medical books.

Assimilation of the practice of acupuncture thus took place within two separate professional groups in Europe: the Jesuits and travelling doctors. Sadly the Jesuits' efforts had little impact on the practice of acupuncture (Hsu 1989). However, the term 'acupuncture' has its origins from Jesuit missionaries as a combination of two Latin words: *acus* (needle) and *punctura* (puncture).

It is worth noting that English translations of Chinese texts can be misleading. Chinese texts are rich in imagery, and compromises may have to be made in translating. For example, the word 'point' in English is not an accurate translation of the Chinese word *xué*. Acupuncture points are usually found in depressions or crevices between bones or sinews, and as such have length, width and depth. Their location is not fixed and are found by palpation; only then are they effective. The term 'point', therefore, does not truly reflect the complex, three-dimensional image of xué (Wilcox 2006).

It was in France that the practice of 'acupuncture' was in vogue at the beginning of the nineteenth century, and from there it spread to other European countries. With a delay of about ten years it spread also to England, Germany and Italy. In England J.M. Churchill wrote two books on acupuncture in

1821 and followed on with a series of case histories. However, this fashion of needling had a short life. Most doctors of the early nineteenth century applied only the so-called 'locus dolendi' mode of treatment where localized pain was treated by the local insertion of needles. Also they felt little or no need to consult Chinese sources (Hsu 1989).

Following the early Western interest in acupuncture in the nineteenth century, it did not return to the public eye until the second half of the twentieth century. For example, the English Acupuncture Association was not formed until 1960 and the British Medical Acupuncture Society not until 1980 as an association of medical practitioners interested in acupuncture.

A significant event occurred in 1971 when Henry A. Kissinger, Secretary of State for President Richard M. Nixon's administration, went to Communist China to prepare for a trip the following year as part of the efforts to re-establish relationships with China. Whilst on the trip, one of the accompanying journalists had an acute appendicitis attack which required an emergency operation.

The journalist, one James Reston of the *New York Times*, suffered from post-operation pain and nausea. To help ease the pain, Chinese doctors used acupuncture in his forearm, which was effective. On his return Reston wrote an article for the *New York Times* where he detailed his own recovery by the use of acupuncture and his other observations of the effectiveness of acupuncture. Acupuncture was further propelled into the minds of the West when Kissinger mentioned the incident during a press conference after the visit to China.

These events sparked the public's curiosity concerning acupuncture and TCM. There was enormous excitement and interest among American doctors and non-physicians alike, with groups of each going to China to seek training and investigate the claims independently.

Prehistoric acupuncture

Acupuncture may have actually already been a practice familiar to ancient Europeans. The mummified remains of the so-called Austrian Iceman, who has come to be known as Otzi, because he was found in a glacier of the Otztal Alps near the border between Austria and Italy, has led to this speculation. What is remarkable about this discovery is that he was perfectly preserved shortly after his death, providing an insight into prehistoric man dating back to 3200 BC.

Initial investigations found that Otzi had 15 groups of simple tattoos marking points on the skin. The tattoos did not appear ornamental, and an acupuncturist was consulted and asked about the possible relationship between the markings and acupuncture points. It was found that 80 per cent of these points corresponded to the acupuncture points used today. Further analysis has confirmed the presence of 61 tattoos divided into 19 groups in various parts of the body.

The tattoos were therefore primarily intended as therapeutic measures rather than as symbols. The points found on Otzi would have been used to treat symptoms of diseases that he seems to have suffered from, such as digestive parasites and osteoarthritis. The purpose of the tattoos is that wherever Otzi went he could go undergo treatment because the points were mapped out for a lay person to use. Further speculation is that a form of bone needle could have been used to stimulate the points similar to the objects found with Otzi.

This discovery indicates that ancient Europeans might have been aware of the practice of acupuncture earlier than had previously been thought. Lars Krutak, a tattoo anthropologist, has uncovered further evidence for medicinal tattooing in Sarawak, Papua New Guinea, again suggesting that practices similar to acupuncture may have already been in existence (Samadelli *et al.* 2015).

Conclusion

Over thousands of years TCM has developed a theoretical and practical approach to the treatment and prevention of many different diseases. TCM has obviously had to deal with a huge range of health conditions, from pandemics to accident and emergency cases. As a result TCM has a vast array of texts and practices describing the diagnosis and treatment of a huge range of disorders. TCM and Oriental medicine is clearly an enormous tradition which has evolved over centuries. It has adapted to different cultures and continues to thrive. The adaptation and integration of acupuncture into Western mainstream healthcare could be considered to be another cultural adaptation.

Eckman (2014, p.34) sums up the arguments from both sides by calling for tolerance: 'Biomedicine gives us one very useful lens to look at health and illness. Oriental medicine provides us with a different, but equally valid and useful lens. Like so many other challenges that face humanity, the solution to this quandary is peaceful coexistence.'

References

Birch, S., and Massutato, K. (1993) *Hara Diagnosis: Reflections on the Sea*. Brookline, MA: Paradigm Press.

Deadman, P. (2014) 'Brief history of qigong.' *Journal of Chinese Medicine 105*, 5–17.

Denmei, S. (2003) *Finding Effective Acupuncture Points*. Washington, DC: Eastland Press.

Eckman, P. (2014) 'Traditional Chinese medicine – science or pseudoscience? A response to Paul Unschuld.' *Journal of Chinese Medicine 104*, 41.

Ergil, K.V., Kramer, E.J., and Ng, A.T. (2002) 'Chinese herbal medicines.' *Western Journal of Medicine 176*, 4, 275–279.

Fixler, M., and Kivity, O. (1988) 'Four styles.' *European Journal of Oriental Medicine 3*, 3.

Hsu, E. (1989) 'Outline of the history of acupuncture.' *Journal of Chinese Medicine 29*, 28–32.

Kan-Wen Ma (2000) 'Acupuncture: its place in the history of Chinese medicine.' *Acupunct. Med. 18*, 88–99.

Kobayashi, A., Uefuji, M., and Yasumo, W. (2010) 'History and progress of Japanese acupuncture.' *Evidence-Based Complementary and Alternative Medicine 7*, 3, 359–365.

Lewith, G. (1982) *Acupuncture: Its Place in Western Medical Science*. London: Thorsons/HarperCollins.

Maciocia, G. (1982) 'History of acupuncture.' *Journal of Chinese Medicine 9*, 3.

Neal, E. (2013) 'Introduction to Neijing classical acupuncture. Part II: Clinical theory.' *Journal of Chinese Medicine 102*, 20–33.

Samadelli, M., Melis, M., Miccoli, M., Vigl, E.R., and Zink, A. (2015) 'Complete mapping of the tattoos of the 5300-year-old Tyrolean Iceman.' *Journal of Cultural Heritage,* January, online.

Sussmutt-Dyckorhoff, C., and Wang, J. (2010) 'China's health care reforms.' *Health International 10*, 54–67.

Wang Ju-Yi and Robertson, J. (2008) *Applied Channel Therapy in Chinese Medicine: Wang Ju-Yi's Lectures on Channel Therapeutics*. Seattle, WA: Eastland Press.

Wang Xue Tai (1984) 'Research into the methods of classical moxibustion.' *Journal of Chinese Medicine 15*, 24–28.

Wilcox, L. (2006) 'What is an acu-moxa point?' *Journal of Chinese Medicine 80*, 5–9.

World Health Organization (2010) *Benchmarks for Training in Tuina*. Geneva: WHO.

Xie, H.R. (2008) 'Discussion on the Qi-passage of channel-collateral system.' *Zhen Ci Yan Jiu 33*, 2, 142–144.

Xinghua, B. (2008) 'How old is acupuncture? Challenging the Neolithic origins.' *Journal of Chinese Medicine 86*, 2, 5–10.

Yuen, J.W.M., Tse, S.H.M., and Yung, J.Y.K. (2012) *Traditional Chinese Herbal Medicine – East Meets West in Validation and Therapeutic Application*. Available at www.intechopen.com/books/recent-advances-in-theories-and-practice-of-chinese-medicine/traditional-chinese-herbal-medicine-east-meets-west-in-validation-and-therapeutic-application, accessed on 2 October 2015.

Zaroff, L. (1999) 'The case of surgery in pre-modern China.' *Journal of Chinese Medicine 59*, online.

Part II

THEORIES AROUND DRY NEEDLING AND TRADITIONAL CHINESE MEDICINE

Chapter 3

Myofascial Pain and Trigger Points

Within clinical practice as manual therapists, we see a large number of patients who present to us daily with pain that arises from muscle and its connective tissue. One understanding is that these patients are suffering with pain caused by myofascial pain syndrome, which is a condition that has been caused by painful trigger points (hence the condition has the acronym MTrPs) situated within the muscles. These can cause pain in a specific spot within a muscle or a painful referral into adjoining areas. Travell and Simons (1999a) state that in one study it is estimated that myofascial pain is a primary cause of regional pain in around 75 per cent of cases. More recently Gerwin (2010) indicates that myofascial trigger points are responsible for, or play a role in, as much as 85 per cent of musculoskeletal pain. Dommerholt, Bron and Franssen (2006) have identified MTrPs with nearly every musculoskeletal pain problem, including radiculopathies, joint dysfunction, disc pathology, tendonitis, craniomandibular dysfunction, migraines, tension-type headaches, carpal tunnel syndrome, whiplash-associated spinal dysfunction, and pelvic pain and other urologic syndromes. Myofascial trigger points are associated with many other pain syndromes, including, for example, post-herpetic neuralgia, complex regional pain syndrome, nocturnal cramps and phantom pain. This list is by no means exhaustive but gives an indication of the widespread prevalence of myofascial pain.

With such a high incidence rate of patients presenting with pain from MTrPs, having a thorough understanding of this condition and its mechanisms of action, and learning effective ways to treat it such as modern acupuncture techniques, are crucial for successful patient management.

Travell and Simons

The trigger point concept (MTrPs) was first coined by Dr Janet Travell. Dr Travell practised as a cardiologist before focusing the majority of her life's work on musculoskeletal pain. Whilst as a cardiologist she noticed that many cases of angina were unaccompanied by any sign of heart problems and were, in fact, spasms of the pectoral muscles causing referred pain mimicking the pain referral patterns of cardiac ischaemia. Dr Travell was also reported to have developed pain in her right shoulder radiating into the right arm, which continued for a year despite numerous investigations into the source of the pain. As no organic source of her pain was found, it was dismissed. It was her own father who eventually cured her pain by injecting procaine into the tender spots; this led to her full recovery (Simons 2003). These experiences and observations led her and long-time partner Dr David Simons to investigate, understand and document myofascial pain. Dr Travell throughout her career attempted to persuade the medical community that the primary cause and contributor to musculoskeletal pain was myofascial syndrome, which was best treated not by surgery or pharmaceutical medicine, but by manual therapies, especially the needle (injections in her case). The culmination of their work was published in *Myofascial Pain and Dysfunction: The Trigger Point Manual*, in two volumes, which have been hailed as the definitive references on myofascial pain and locating trigger points. In these publications trigger points and their corresponding zones of radiating pain were recorded and illustrated in virtually every muscle of the body. Travell was also appointed as the White House physician from 1961 to 1965 due to her curing of John F. Kennedy's long-term back pain. Travell coined the term 'myofascial' to describe the involvement of both muscle and fascia, and 'trigger point' to convey the notion that pain radiates from one site to another, often at some distance. It their systematic documentation of trigger points that manual therapists owe much to, and is responsible for many of the trigger point charts that are seen in clinics.

Early historical observations

J.H. Kellgren published two important papers that inspired Travell to investigate the myofascial pain phenomenon. The first, in 1938, was entitled 'Observations on referred pain arising from muscle'; and the second, in 1939, was entitled 'On the distribution of referred pain arising from deep somatic structures with charts of segmental pain areas'. In his experiments Kellgren injected saline solution into healthy volunteers' muscles and recorded that pain resulting from the injection produced pain that was distant from the injection site. From these early observations many other physicians continued to map these referral patterns and confirmed the hypothesis that pain can be referred in distinct reliable and reproducible patterns. Another key factor was that injecting anaesthetic into trigger points or hyper-irritable areas relieved this type of pain, and this eventually led to the discovery that using acupuncture needles was safer than, and just as effective as, hypodermic needles.

Definition of myofascial trigger points

Myofascial pain is a regional muscle pain disorder characterized by localized muscle tenderness and pain and is frequently the cause of persistent pain. Myofascial pain has accompanying sensory, motor and autonomic symptoms. Evaluation of myofascial pain includes locating the trigger points and muscles involved as well as recognition of other contributing factors. Manual therapy and acupuncture are tools to deactivate MTrPs whilst restoring the muscle to its normal length and full joint range of motion with exercises and stretches.

MTrPs are characterized by 'a hypersensitive spot, usually within a taut band of skeletal muscle or in the muscle's fascia, they can have strong focal points of tenderness, a few millimeters in diameter, and be found at multiple sites in muscle tissue' (Travell and Simons 1999b, p.34). Biopsy tests have further found that these trigger points are not only hyper-irritable but also electrically active muscle spindles in general muscle tissue (Hubbard 1996, 1998; Hubbard and Berkoff 1993).

A good example of a common trigger point many therapists encounter can be found in the trapezius muscles, as these muscles help to maintain posture, and MTrPs in this area are a common cause of non-specific and mechanical neck pain. Equally, they are one of the foremost pain-presenting complaints seen by manual therapists, especially in the upper trapezius (Rickards 2006).

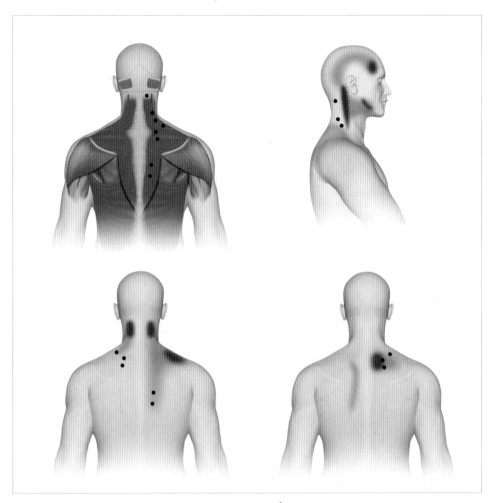

Figure 3.1 Trapezius muscle trigger points

Although Travell and Simons may have coined the term 'trigger points', it seems that traditional acupuncturists have in fact been working with MTrPs from the very start, as it has been shown that over 70 per cent of MTrPs correspond to acupuncture points when used to treat pain (Dorsher 2009). This is why there is such similarity between traditional and modern acupuncture techniques when treating patients who present with myofascial pain symptoms.

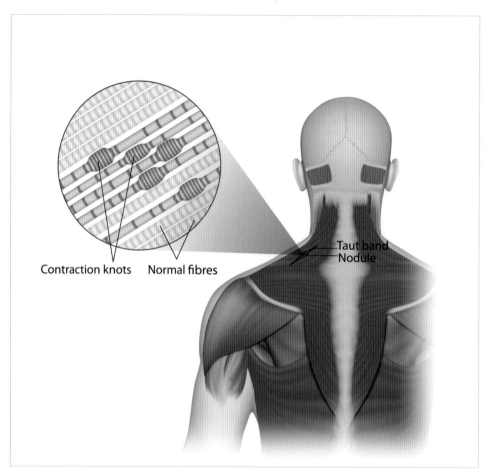

Contraction knots   Normal fibres

Taut band
Nodule

Figure 3.2 Trigger point complex

MTrPs can be further broken down into active and latent.

Active trigger points

An active MTrP is, as mentioned above, a hypersensitive area which 'causes a pattern of referred pain at rest/or on motion', which is clinically associated with a local twitch response (Travell and Simons 1999b, p.40).

Latent trigger points

These are still areas of hypersensitivity and include the same presentation as previously described; however, they only refer pain when palpated, as opposed to active MTrPs that exhibit pain and referral without palpation (Travell and Simons 1999b, p.59).

Clinical presentation

Common characteristics of both latent and active trigger points (Menses and Simons 2001) are the following:

- An MTrP has a clear and consistent pain pattern, and a pain referral pattern to its given location on a referral zone map is outlined by Travell and Simons' research.

- MTrPs can arise in response to acute and chronic overloading, or repetitive overuse of the muscle in which it occurs.

- MTrPs contribute to motor dysfunction by causing increased muscle tension.

- MTrPs cause weakness and a limited range of motion.

- The intensity and extent of the pain depends on the degree of irritability of the MTrPs and not on the size or location of the muscle.

- MTrPs can disturb the proprioceptive, nociceptive and autonomic functions of the affected anatomical region.

As you can see, both active and latent trigger points can present in a number of different ways within a patient's symptoms, from large referral areas of pain, muscle weakness, inhibition, increased motor dysfunction, muscular imbalances, spasm and an altering of motor recruitment (Lucas, Polus and Rich 2004). Therefore a full case history has to be taken with each patient to ensure that all possible causes of the pain and possible red flags have been ruled out prior to a diagnosis of MTrPs.

There are alternative theories as to what causes patients to feel pain in these MTrP locations, and just as research shows that meridian acupuncture points can mirror trigger points, so the distribution of pain that is being referred from these MTrPs has a close relationship with the course of the peripheral nerves. It is also shown that pain from myofascial pain syndrome is also similar to nerve trunk pain, which is an example of somatic referred pain. One theory is that, rather than the MTrPs being the primary source of this increased sensitivity to pain, myofascial pain syndrome is better explained as a secondary hyperalgesia of peripheral neural origin (Quinter 1994).

The exact pathological processes and aetiology of MTrPs are, as yet, to be confirmed, with both imaging and histological studies said to be inconclusive (Huguenin 2004). There are a number of theories looking at the mechanisms of action for the causes of MTrPs, one of which looks at MTrPs originating at the dysfunctional endplates of the muscle fibres (Simons *et al.* 1999); this may be enhanced by contributing factors such as:

- acute/chronic overload of a muscle

- overloading of the antagonist muscle – therefore causing muscular tension

- a muscle becoming irritated due to its location in the referral path of another MTrP.

More recent research suggests that MTrPs are a combination of these contributing factors plus the presence of 'neuromuscular lesions that form part of a neurological loop that affects and is affected by the CNS' (Lucas *et al.* 2004, p.162).

Theories and research into this topic will continue to cause necessary debate amongst therapists from all therapeutic disciplines, but whether we subscribe to traditional points, trigger points or other theories, the use of acupuncture, medical acupuncture or dry needling has been shown to be an effective way to treat muscular pain.

Muscle contraction

Muscle contraction is triggered by acetylcholine (ACh) release in the neuromuscular junction. ACh binds to receptors on the muscle membrane, and the resulting potential triggers calcium release. The calcium binds to troponin, which slides tropomyosin off the actin-binding sites. Once the neural command has ended, acetylcholinesterase (AChE) enters the synaptic cleft and breaks down ACh.

The integrated trigger point hypothesis

The integrated trigger point hypothesis integrates a number of perpetuating factors into one thesis. The theory starts at the synaptic cleft where acetylcholine is abnormally released. This increases the number of miniature endplate potentials producing endplate noise and sustained depolarization of the membrane of the muscle fibre. The continuous depolarization causes the release and inadequate uptake of calcium ions from local sarcoplasmic reticulum and produces muscle shortening of sarcomeres. It is further suggested that, in addition to motor neuron irritability, during contraction myosin filaments get stuck in the gel-like substance titin in the Z-band, preventing the sarcomere from returning to resting length. Constant shortening of the muscle results in muscle tissue ischaemia restricting local blood vessels, thus reducing the oxygen and nutritional supply. Without oxidative ability, there is a shortage in ATP. The shortage of ATP in MTrPs also contributes to the sustained contraction, and the muscle is not able to break down actin–myosin bonds – an 'energy crisis'. This shortening causes a loss of oxygen and nutrient supply in the presence of an increased metabolic demand, hence the energy crisis. This energy crisis releases sensitizing substances which cause pain, interfere with autonomic and sensory nerves and send autonomic stimulation back to the neuromuscular junction to restart the cycle and further aggravate the problem.

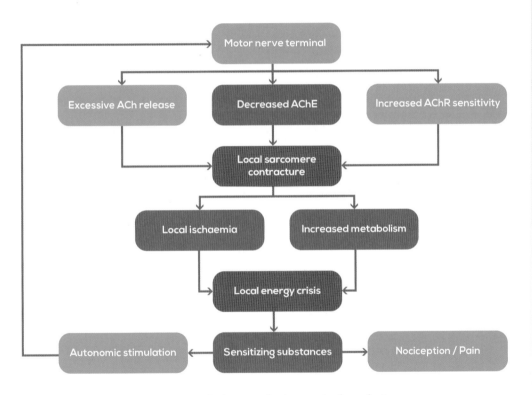

Figure 3.3 The integrated trigger point hypothesis

Locating MTrPs

Currently a diagnosis of myofascial pain syndrome (MPS) requires the therapist to palpate for the identification of at least one clinically relevant MTrP. However, very few comparable, high-quality studies currently exist from which to draw firm conclusions regarding the robustness of MTrPs' examination (Myburgh *et al.* 2011).

Imaging such as ultrasounds and the MRIs of MTrPs have shown to have no diagnostic relevance in the locating of active or latent MTrPs. This raises a problem for the manual therapist: how do you locate an MTrP in order to accurately insert an acupuncture needle into it or into the area around it? For this book we will focus on the key skill of all therapists, which is their palpation – their ability to accurately work with the tissues of the body to identify areas of pain; and using the techniques shown within this book, successfully treat them with medical acupuncture/dry needling. There is no 'X marks the spot' with MTrPs, as every patient is different, but this book and its technique guides give the therapist a clear area of where they need to palpate in order to decide where to place the needle.

Some clinical indications to aid therapists in the identification of MTrPs are the following (Hong and Simons 1998):

- Compression of an MTrP may elicit local and/or referred pain that is similar to a patient's usual clinical complaint (pain recognition) or may aggravate the existing pain.

- Snapping palpation (compression across the muscle fibres rapidly) may elicit a local twitch response, which is a brisk contraction of the muscle fibres in or around the taut band.

- Restricted range of stretch, and increased sensitivity to stretch, of muscle fibres in a taut band may cause tightness of the involved muscle.

- Patients with MTrPs may have associated localized autonomic phenomena, including vasoconstriction, pilomotor response, ptosis and hypersecretion.

Once a suspected trigger is found, pressure can be applied to determine if it is active. Moderate but sustained palpation of an MTrP tends to accentuate the pain of an active MTrP.

The following questions asked on application of pressure are:

1. 'Does this hurt?'

2. 'Is this causing pain anywhere else?'

3. 'Is this the pain you have been experiencing?'

If the answers to these questions are all 'yes', this is an active myofascial trigger point. (Refer to Chapter 8 for a more detailed insight into locating MTrPs.)

Local twitch response

An indication of locating an MTrP and also of effective needling technique, or that a treatment will have a positive outcome, can be seen when a muscle exhibits a local twitch response (LTR). This is a sudden and sometimes quite large contraction within that specific muscle, and can shock both patient and practitioner. The LTR is a valuable sign for the practitioner, as it confirms the presence of an MTrP, and studies have shown that a transient burst of electromyographic (EMG) activity can be clearly recorded from taut band fibres when an LTR is elicited by snapping palpation of an MTrP (Hong *et al.* 1997). The LTR has a direct relationship within traditional acupuncture and the theory of deqi, which is usually translated as 'to obtain or grasp the qi when needling an acupuncture point'.

LTRs are effectively a spinal cord reflex elicited by stimulating the sensitive site in an MTrP. It has been shown to be linked with a decrease in endplate noise (Hong 1994), and post-LTR a marked reduction in the concentration of many chemicals situated within a muscle that can be implicated in nociception (Shah *et al.* 2005). These effects are likely to lead to the reduction in the sensitivity and myofascial pain intensity.

It is also indicated that if a muscle produces a significant number of LTRs when stimulated by an acupuncture needle, then this is due to an increased chemical irritation of that muscle's nociceptors (Hong *et al.* 1997). Clinical experience has shown that muscles that have hypersensitive MTrPs will commonly produce a greater number of LTRs when stimulated with acupuncture than areas that are not dysfunctional.

Radiculopathy and chronic pain

Radiculopathy is a condition due to a compressed nerve or nerves in the spine that can cause pain, numbness, tingling or weakness along the course of the nerve. Radiculopathy can occur in any part of the spine, but it is most common in the lumbar and cervical region. The dysfunction and damage to the nerves is called a neuropathy. Radiculopathy can be thought of as deep myofascial pain of paraspinal origin.

Dr Chan Gunn is recognized as establishing a system for treating chronic pain due to radiculopathy. He is the founder and president of the Institute for the Study and Treatment of Pain in Vancouver, British Columbia, Canada. Dr Gunn created the technique of Intramuscular Stimulation (IMS), which is a diagnostic and treatment model for myofascial pain of neuropathic origin. It works by stimulating spinal reflexes that reverse muscle contractures (shortened muscles) through the use of fine, flexible acupuncture-style needles.

Radiculopathy is sometimes referred to as the short muscle syndrome. With increased muscle contraction, this affects the autonomic nervous system (ANS) by impinging nerves at the nerve root. The nerve impingement reduces the flow of motor impulses throughout the nerve pathway. According to Cannon and Rosenblueth's Law of Denervation, a reduction of motor impulses through a nerve pathway produces disuse sensitivity and abnormal behaviour within the receptor organ or tissue. The Law of Denervation also claims that the function and integrity of all innervated structures are reliant on normal nerve functioning. Due to muscle contraction, the flow of proteins, hormones, enzymes, neurotransmitters and electrical input along nerve fibres is blocked. The innervated structures such as muscles, glands and neural pathways are now deprived of the essential materials for normal functioning, resulting in abnormal sensitivity and dysfunction (Christie 2007).

Radiculopathy also influences other tissues throughout the entire dermatome by reducing the flow of motor impulses at the nerve root. Nerve impingement and radiculopathy also influence distal pain by elevating acetylcholine and adrenaline levels throughout the pathways, thereby increasing susceptibility to extremity muscular contraction (Weiner 2001).

Continuous muscle shortening causes mechanical strain on other structures such as tendons, ligaments and joints. Increased mechanical pressure can cause further problems such as tendonitis, bursitis, enthesopathy – thickening of tendons to their attachments (e.g. semispinalis capitis at the occiput) – degenerative arthritis and increased disc degeneration.

Gunn often referred to paraspinal shortening as 'the invisible lesion', as it cannot be seen on diagnostic imaging and requires examination by deep needling, often felt as hard resistance when a shortened paraspinal muscle is reached (Gunn 1996).

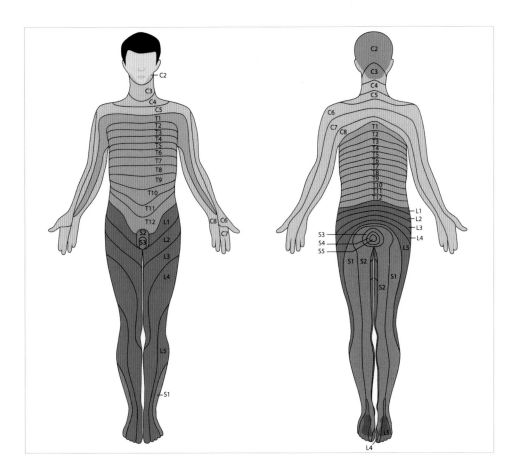

Figure 3.4 Dermatome Chart

As with all patients, treatment includes taking a detailed history (especially dermatomal and myotomal distributions), examination, palpation and observation. Gunn emphasized some key physical findings when examining a patient, but as radiculopathy involves the paraspinal muscles then these must be individually palpated (Gunn 2002):

- Palpation may include deep needle of the affected/suspected area for contractures.

- Affected regions may have paraspinal muscles and spinous processes that are more prominent and tender on palpation.

- In the cervical spine, posterior and lateral neck creases at segmental levels indicate involvement at that level.

- Resistance to needle penetration is a sign that the level is affected. Needling may be repeated by lifting and thrusting the needle until such resistance diminishes, possibly over several treatments.

- There may be loss of joint range or pain caused by the mechanical effects of muscle shortening.

- There may be sensory alteration: hyperalgesia – increased sensitivity to pain.

- There may be autonomic features.

- Affected areas may feel cold due to vasoconstriction.

- The affected area may exhibit excess perspiration.

- There may be piloerection or goosebumps over the affected area.

- There may be excess fluid in the subcutaneous tissues, as in trophedema: oedema in hands and feet, dermatomal hair loss, inadequate or faulty nutrition of skin and nails due to poor nerve supply.

- Possible tests to confirm autonomic dysfunctions include the matchstick test, the skin rolling test and the red line test (there are others, but these are simple and quick to perform).

- Treatment aims to reduce muscle shortening by the same mechanisms as standard needling for myofascial pain.

Articular and joint dysfunction

Travell and Simons (1999a) categorized articular dysfunction as one of three major categories of MSK pain, being either a primary or aggravating factor of myofascial pain. They were in later years influenced by osteopathic and chiropractic medicine – practitioners such as Irvin Korr and Karl Lewitt helped form their later opinions on this subject, and the second editions of their books contained updated information on the subject.

When both an articular dysfunction and muscular problem are present, then obviously they both need treating. The two conditions can aggravate each other. Myofascial pain increases muscle tension and may create stresses on the joints that predispose them to articular dysfunction. The articular dysfunction is thought to disturb the motor, sensory and autonomic nervous system just as with myofascial pain and therefore leads to muscular hyperactivity, which in turn causes or exacerbates myofascial pain (Clark *et al.* 2012).

Manipulation and mobilization techniques are thought to reduce the excitability of the muscle spindle afferents and so reduce reflexive contractile activity. Clark *et al.* (2012) propose that manipulation and mobilization work by reducing nociceptive input, which in turn reduces excitatory input to the γ-motoneurons, thereby normalizing the excitability of the stretch reflex. This decreased stretch reflex response, coupled with the reduced nociceptive input, lessens excitatory input to the α-motoneuron pool, ultimately decreasing muscle activity. Post-treatment there is an increased range of motion at the joint, helping to restore normal tissue functioning, which encourages normal movement.

Peripheral and central sensitization

Potentially injury-causing stimuli are detected by nociceptors, which are specialized nerves that are found in the skin, muscle and viscera. Nociceptors respond to tissue damage and can cause a sensation of pain when they are activated (Woolf 2010). This process is adaptive in that pain protects us from further damage. Maladaptive pain, in contrast, is an expression of the pathologic operation of the nervous system; it is pain as disease, and even light touch can be considered as a noxious stimulus in extreme cases (Woolf 2006). Both peripheral sensitization and central sensitization have common characteristics in their response:

- Thresholds are lowered so that stimuli that would normally not produce pain now begin to do so (allodynia).

- Responsiveness is increased, so that noxious stimuli produce an exaggerated and prolonged pain (hyperalgesia).

- Pain is no longer protective and serves no purpose. Changes in pain associated with tissue damage and/or other pain triggers result in prolonged modulation of the somatosensory system, with increased responsiveness of both peripheral and central pain pathways. Ongoing pain can also be absent from a trigger or stimulus.

Peripheral sensitization

Woolf (2006, p.14) describes peripheral sensitization as 'a reduction in threshold and an increase in responsiveness of the peripheral ends of nociceptors, the high-threshold peripheral sensory neurons that transfer input from peripheral targets (skin, muscle, joints and the viscera) through peripheral nerves to the central nervous system (spinal cord and brainstem)'.

Tissue damage leads to a cascade of inflammatory substances being released, including potassium ions, substance P, bradykinin and prostaglandins. These substances may induce a sensitization of peripheral receptors with changes in the response characteristics of primary afferent fibres. They may activate normally inactive or 'silent' nociceptors. Activation of latent trigger points may be part of this process (Latremoliere and Woolf 2009).

Acute nociceptive pain is that physiological sensation of hurt that results from the activation of nociceptive pathways by peripheral stimuli of sufficient intensity to lead to or to threaten tissue damage (noxious stimuli). Nociception, the detection of noxious stimuli, is a protective process that helps prevent injury by both generating a reflex withdrawal from the stimulus and as a sensation so unpleasant that it results in complex behavioural strategies to avoid further contact with such stimuli (Latremoliere and Woolf 2009).

Central sensitization

Woolf (2010, p.18) describes central sensitization as 'an increase in the excitability of neurons within the central nervous system, so that normal inputs begin to produce abnormal responses'.

Central hypersensitivity has been documented in a number of conditions including osteoarthritis, tension-type headache, temporomandibular joint pain, endometriosis post-mastectomy and visceral pain. Again the pain is no longer protective and serves no purpose.

Central sensitization is now thought to be the process behind referred pain associated with myofascial pain. The prolonged afferent nociceptive input may induce a reversible increase in the excitability of central sensory neurons combined with an expansion of the receptive field, resulting in any peripheral stimulus activating a higher number of dorsal horn neurons with an increased sensitivity to pain. Other theories propose that prolonged muscle tension stretches specific portions of this fascia, activating pain receptors within the tissue. This may further enhance the nociceptive input in central sensitization.

A good example is the trapezius muscle, which has low mechanical receptors and therefore a lower pain threshold than other muscles. Repeated stimulation (such as the upper crossed syndrome in office workers, for example) results in short-lasting pain, with the possibility of central sensitization due to the continuous nociceptive input. This may explain the high frequency of chronic pain at the neck and shoulder region often seen by physical therapists.

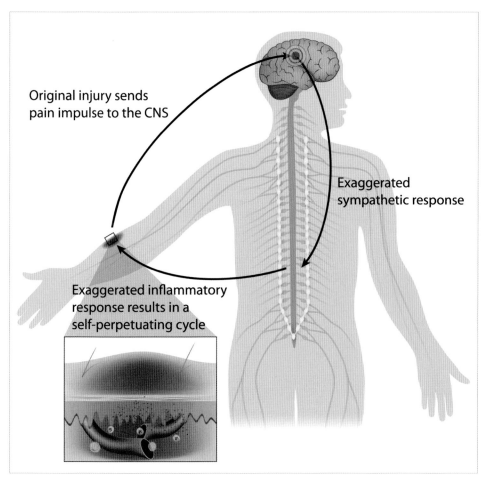

Original injury sends pain impulse to the CNS

Exaggerated sympathetic response

Exaggerated inflammatory response results in a self-perpetuating cycle

Figure 3.5 Complex regional pain syndrome

Central sensitization is now recognized as part of visceral pain where an increased sensitivity occurs in the viscera following an injury or inflammation of an internal organ. The implications are far-reaching, from post-operations to ongoing dysmenorrhoea and IBS being factors to consider when taking a case history.

Detecting hypersensitivity can be troublesome, but simple quantitative sensory tests may act as a guide. Typically, a standardized and quantifiable sensory stimulus is applied at a peripheral tissue. The stimulus intensity is increased gradually until the subject perceives the stimulus as painful (Woolf 2010). If suspected in a patient, then use the 'less is more' approach to begin with, so as not to over-stimulate.

Autonomic nervous system disturbances

The major researchers into myofascial trigger points, Travell and Simons (Simons *et al.* 1999; Travell and Simons 1999b), have shown that trigger points interfere with the autonomic nervous systems in numerous ways. This includes abnormal secretions in the areas where the trigger points exist, muscle cramps, abnormal motor function (eye twitching, for example), excessive sweating, pilomotor activity, changes in skin temperature, lacrimation and salivation. Autonomic nervous system disturbances caused by a trigger point will improve once it has been removed.

Some common clinical examples are (adapted from Chaitow and Fritz 2006):

- appendicitis-like pain, usually during the premenstrual phase of the cycle (the trigger point may be located at the lower right margin of the rectus abdominis muscle)

- calf cramps, fasciculation (gastrocnemius)

- proprioceptive disturbances, dizziness/vertigo (suboccipitals)

- excessive lacrimation (trigger points in facial muscles)

- shortness of breath (scalenes, levator scapula)

- cardiac arrhythmias (trigger points in the pectoralis major in particular)

- conjunctival reddening (trigger points in the cervical or facial muscles)

- dermatographia (trigger points referring to an area where dermatographia is noted)

- diarrhoea, dysmenorrhoea, diminished gastric motility, bloating (trigger points in abdominals, i.e. rectus abdominis)

- excessive maxillary sinus secretion (trigger points in facial muscles – often the sternocleidomastoid is involved)

- vasoconstriction and headache (trigger points lie in the cervical or facial musculature).

When taking the patient's history, it is important to establish, if possible, the order of problems to determine whether the trigger point is the primary or secondary cause of pain and dysfunction. Autonomic disturbances may be due to visceral problems. Visceral pain is often felt in places remote from the location of the affected organ. This is known as 'referred pain' and it is often very useful in the diagnosis of diseases of the internal organs. For instance, not all internal organs are sensitive to pain, and some can be damaged quite extensively without the person feeling a thing. Refer to Figure 3.6 for further information when considering visceral damage and dysfunction.

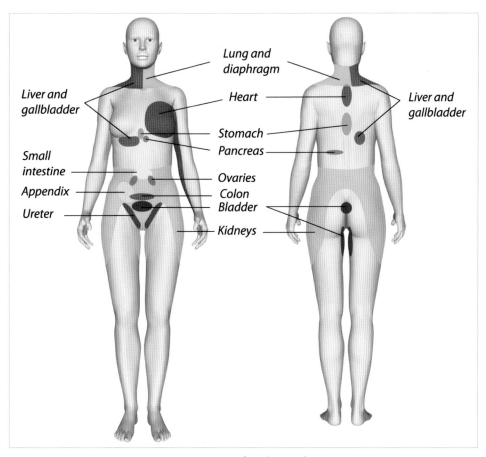

Figure 3.6 Referred pain chart

Non-structural perpetuating factors: biological, nutritional, genetic and other non-mechanical factors

Lederman (2011) claims that manual and physical therapists often use a postural-structural-biomechanical (PSB) model to ascertain the causes of various musculoskeletal conditions. It is believed that postural deviations, body asymmetries and pathomechanics are the predisposing/maintaining factors for many musculoskeletal conditions. The PSB model also plays an important role in clinical assessment and management, including the choice of manual techniques and the exercise prescribed.

However, focusing on a single factor may be ineffective and multiple factors may need to be considered, so taking a comprehensive detailed history is crucial and laboratory examinations may be required. The role of the practitioner is to identify the underlying cause or causes of persistent or chronic muscle pain in order to develop a specific treatment plan which may involve one or more treatment options. Biological, nutritional and genetic factors must be considered when patients fail to respond to manual therapy or do not make a full recovery as expected. Widespread muscle pain is more likely to be metabolic and therefore needs to be clinically recognized, tested and treated. Any deficiency that interferes with the energy supply of muscle is likely to aggravate MTrPs.

Vitamin inadequacies lead to:

- impaired cell metabolism and function

- decreased synthesis of neurotransmitters and DNA

- impaired collagen synthesis and reduced nerve and muscle function

- increased irritability of trigger points and nerves.

The following are some key examples to consider.

Vitamin D deficiency

Close to 90 per cent of patients with chronic musculoskeletal pain may have vitamin D deficiency. Vitamin D plays an important role in skeletal development, bone health maintenance and neuromuscular functioning. Because the signs and symptoms of vitamin D deficiency are insidious or non-specific, it often goes unrecognized and untreated (Bordelon, Ghetu and Langan 2009).

Figures show that up to a quarter of the population has low levels of vitamin D in their blood and the majority of pregnant women do not take vitamin D supplements. In the UK around 1 in 5 adults, and around 1 in 6 children, may have low vitamin D status – an estimated 10 million people in total. This can be clearly seen over the past few years, with the increase of rickets in British Asian children and recent immigrants to the UK, particularly in second generation black African or Caribbean parents from socially and economically deprived areas.

Vitamin D is naturally obtained through exposure to sunlight and from foods such as oily fish, eggs, fortified fat spreads and some fortified breakfast cereals. But it is difficult to get enough from food alone. In musculoskeletal pain it is a key component that determines neuromuscular functioning. Plotnikoff and Quigley (2003) found that 89 per cent of subjects with chronic musculoskeletal pain were deficient in vitamin D2. Vitamin D deficiency is associated with musculoskeletal pain, loss of type II muscle fibres, and proximal muscle atrophy.

The deficiency state is easily corrected, but it takes up to six months of replacement to reverse changes caused by deficiency states. The following risk factors have been identified:

- age over 65 years

- breastfed exclusively without vitamin D supplementation

- dark skin, for example people of African, African-Caribbean and South Asian origin, because their bodies are not able to make as much vitamin D

- insufficient sunlight exposure, for example those who cover their skin for cultural reasons, who are housebound or who are confined indoors for long periods

- medication use that alters vitamin D metabolism (e.g. anticonvulsants, glucocorticoids)

- obesity (body mass index greater than 30 kg per m^2)

- sedentary lifestyle

- all pregnant and breastfeeding women, especially teenagers and young women

- infants and young children under five years of age.

Tague *et al.* (2011) hypothesized that vitamin D deficiency contributes to muscle hypersensitivity through direct effects on sensory nociception neurons. Their other findings in animal studies show that four weeks of a vitamin D-deficient diet produces muscle mechanical hypersensitivity and balance deficits.

Iron deficiency

Sources vary, but estimates are that roughly 10–15 per cent of people with widespread myofascial pain may have some form of iron deficiency. Iron is essential for the generation of energy within muscles, and a deficiency of iron creates an energy crisis in muscle by limiting an energy-producing reaction, leading and/or contributing to myofascial pain. Iron deficiency is reversed by the oral and intravenous route of medication and supplements. It is more prevalent in women who have heavy periods, are pregnant or are menopausal.

Magnesium and zinc deficiency

Your body has a limited ability to store zinc and operates within a narrow margin to supply all of your health needs. However, zinc is poorly consumed with a large percentage of diets. The same is true of magnesium, with most daily intakes being below the recommended daily amount. Both can contribute to myofascial pain.

Hormonal dysfunction

Hypothyroidism occurs when you have insufficient amounts of thyroid hormone or when you have thyroid hormone resistance. As a result, your body cannot maintain normal metabolism, and your ability to convert tyrosine to dopamine, norepinephrine and epinephrine is impaired. Common clinical signs of hypothyroidism, including myofascial pain, are fatigue, hair loss, weight gain, dry skin, hair and eyes, and delayed deep tendon reflexes.

Growth hormone deficiency

Growth hormone is essential for normal linear growth and the attainment of an adult mature height. It also plays an important role in cartilage growth and the attainment of normal bone mass. Suboptimal growth hormone secretion, leading to a state of adult growth hormone deficiency, may occur in the setting of chronic inflammatory disease, chronic corticosteroid use, and fibromyalgia (Bennett 2005). Other clinical signs to consider include (Bennett 2005):

- *joint involvement* – cartilage hyperplasia, synovial proliferation, secondary osteoarthritis, joint hypermobility, capsular thickening, bursal enlargement

- *muscle involvement* – muscle enlargement, proximal weakness, myalgias, muscle cramping

- *nerve involvement* – carpal tunnel syndrome, palpable peripheral nerves, peripheral neuropathy.

Autoimmune diseases

Patients with genetic autoimmune diseases will often seek treatment for severe pain that has developed. This class of diseases includes such painful conditions as ankylosing spondylitis, Behçet's disease, Ehlers-Danlos syndrome, Marfan syndrome and Schmidt's syndrome. These conditions and other connective tissue disorders can often be dismissed – misdiagnosed as fibromyalgia and myofascial pain. The key is in both history and examination. Patients will often have a history of illnesses and sickness in childhood.

Lyme disease is a bacterial infection spread to humans by infected ticks. Many patients who are initially diagnosed with myopathies, neuropathies or arthropathies later prove to have Lyme disease. It is estimated there are 2000 to 3000 new cases of Lyme disease in England and Wales each year. Recently, the Centers for Disease Control and Prevention (CDC) dramatically increased the estimate of the annual number of new cases of Lyme disease in the United States from 30,000 to 300,000 (Kuehn 2013).

Other

Deficiencies in vitamins B1, B6 and C have also been associated with diffuse muscle pain.

Reasons why myofascial therapy fails

There can be a number of reasons why therapy fails to resolve myofascial pain:

- primary trigger point(s) not deactivated

- lack of skill in palpation, detection and deactivation

- treatment is being directed at a secondary myofascial pain syndrome

- perpetuating factors are present, including any physical, chemical or psychological factors that have not been addressed.

References

Bennett, R. (2005) 'Growth hormone in musculoskeletal pain states.' *Current Pain and Headache Reports 9*, 5, 331–338.

Bordelon, P., Ghetu, M., and Langan, R. (2009) 'Recognition and management of vitamin D deficiency.' *American Family Physician 80*, 8, 841–846.

Chaitow, L., and Fritz, S. (2006) *A Massage Therapist's Guide to Understanding, Locating and Treating Myofascial Trigger Points.* Edinburgh: Churchill Livingstone.

Christie, D. (2007) 'The enigma of chronic pain.' *MUMJ 4*, 1, 69.

Clark, B.C., Thomas, J.S., Walkowski, S.A., and Howell, J.N. (2012) 'The biology of manual therapies.' *J. Am. Osteopath. Assoc. 112*, 9, 617–629.

Dommerholt, J., Bron, C., and Franssen, J. (2006) 'Myofascial trigger points: an evidence-informed review.' *Journal of Manual & Manipulative Therapy 14*, 4, 203–221.

Dorsher, P.T. (2009) 'Myofascial referred-pain data provide physiologic evidence of acupuncture meridians.' *J. Pain 10*, 7, 723–731.

Gerwin, R. (2010) 'Myofascial pain syndrome: here we are; where must we go?' *J. Musculoskel. Pain 18*, 4, 329–347.

Gunn, C. (1996) *The Gunn Approach to the Treatment of Chronic Pain* (second edition). Edinburgh: Churchill Livingstone.

Gunn, C. (2002) *Prespondylosis and Some Pain Syndromes Following Denervation Supersensitivity.* Institute for the Study and Treatment of Pain. Available at www.istop.org/papers/prespondylosis.htm, accessed on 17 July 2015.

Hong, C.Z. (1994) 'Lidocaine injection versus dry needling to myofascial trigger point: the importance of the local twitch response.' *Am. J. Phys. Med. Rehabil. 73*, 256–263.

Hong, C.Z., and Simons, D.G. (1998) 'Pathophysiologic and electrophysiologic mechanisms of myofascial trigger points.' *Arch. Phys. Med. Rehabil. 79*, 863–872.

Hong, C.Z., Kuan, T.S., Chen, J.T., *et al.* (1997) 'Referred pain elicited by palpation and by needling of myofascial trigger points: a comparison.' *Arch. Phys. Med Rehabil. 78*, 957–960.

Hubbard, D.R. (1996) 'Chronic and recurrent muscle pain: pathophysiology and treatment, and review of pharmacologic studies.' *J. Musculoskeletal Pain 4*, 123–143.

Hubbard, D.R. (1998) 'Persistent muscular pain: approaches to relieving trigger points.' *J. Musculoskeletal Medicine 15*, 16–26.

Hubbard, D.R., and Berkoff, G. (1993) 'Myofascial trigger points show spontaneous needle EMG activity.' *Spine 18*, 1803–1807.

Huguenin, L.K. (2004) 'Myofascial trigger points: the current evidence.' *Physical Therapy in Science 5*, 1, 2–12.

Kellgren, J.H. (1938) 'Observations on referred pain arising from muscle.' *Clinical Science 3*, 175–190.

Kellgren, J.H. (1939) 'On the distribution of referred pain arising from deep somatic structures with charts of segmental pain areas.' *Clinical Science 4*, 35–46.

Kuehn, B.M. (2013) 'CDC estimates 300,000 US cases of Lyme disease annually.' *JAMA 310*, 11, 1110.

Latremoliere, A., and Woolf, C. (2009) 'Central sensitization: a generator of pain hypersensitivity by central neural plasticity.' *Journal of Pain 10*, 9, 895–926.

Lederman, J. (2011) 'The fall of the postural-structural-biomechanical model in manual and physical therapies: exemplified by lower back pain.' *J. Bodyw. Mov. Ther. 15*, 2, 131–138.

Lucas, K.R., Polus, B.I., and Rich, P.A. (2004) 'Latent myofascial trigger points: effects on muscle activation and movement efficiency.' *J. Bodyw. Mov. Ther. 8*, 160–166.

Menses, S., and Simons, D.G. (2001) *Muscle Pain: Understanding Its Nature, Diagnosis, and Treatment.* Baltimore: Lippincott Williams & Wilkins.

Myburgh, C., Lauridsen, H.H., Larsen, A.H., and Hartvigsen, J. (2011) 'Standardized manual palpation of myofascial trigger points in relation to neck/shoulder pain: the influence of clinical experience on inter-examiner reproducibility.' *Manual Therapy 16*, 2, 136–140.

Plotnikoff, G.A., and Quigley, J.M. (2003) 'Prevalence of severe hypovitaminosis D in patients with persistent, nonspecific musculoskeletal pain.' *Mayo Clin. Proc. 78*, 12, 1463–1470.

Quinter, J.L. (1994) 'Referred pain of peripheral nerve origin: an alternative to the "myofascial pain" construct.' *Clin. J. Pain 10*, 3, 243–251.

Rickards, L.D. (2006) 'The effectiveness of non-invasive treatments for active myofascial trigger point pain: a systematic review of the literature.' *International Journal of Osteopathic Medicine 9*, 4, 120–136.

Shah, J.P., Phillips, T.M., Danoff, J.V., and Gerber, L.H. (2005) 'An in-vivo microanalytical technique for measuring the local biochemical milieu of human skeletal muscle.' *J. Appl. Physiol. 99*, 1977–1984.

Simons, D. (2003) 'Cardiology and myofascial trigger points: Janet G. Travell's contribution.' *Tex. Heart Inst. J. 30*, 1, 3–7.

Tague, S.E., Clarke, G.L., Winter, M.K., McCarson, K.E., Wright, D.E., and Smith, P.G. (2011) 'Vitamin D deficiency promotes skeletal muscle hypersensitivity and sensory hyperinnervation.' *Journal of Neuroscience 31*, 39, 13728–13738.

Travell, J.G., and Simons, L.S. (1999a) *Myofascial Pain and Dysfunction: Upper Half of Body Volume 1: The Trigger Point Manual* (second edition). Baltimore: Lippincott Williams & Wilkins.

Travell, J.G., and Simons, D.G. (1999b) *Myofascial Pain and Dysfunction: Lower Extremities Volume 2: The Trigger Point Manual* (second edition). Baltimore: Lippincott Williams & Wilkins.

Weiner, R. (2001) *Pain Management: A Practical Guide for Clinicians* (sixth edition). Sonora, CA: American Academy of Pain Management.

Woolf, C. (2006) 'Pain: moving from symptom control toward mechanism-specific pharmacologic management.' *Ann. Intern. Med. 140*, 441–451.

Woolf, C. (2010) 'Central sensitization: implications for the diagnosis and treatment of pain.' *Pain 152*, 3 Suppl., S2–15.

Chapter 4

Physiological Mechanism of Acupuncture in Pain Control

Introduction

Acupuncture is one of the oldest forms of alternative medicine. It involves insertion of fine needles through the skin at certain points on the body surface for a therapeutic effect. The term acupuncture derives from two Latin roots, *acus*, meaning 'needle', and *punctura*, meaning 'to puncture' (Pyne and Shenker 2008). The practice has many different methods and forms worldwide. In the West, two main approaches are widely used: traditional and Western medical.

Traditional acupuncture has its origins in ancient Chinese philosophy and has been a fundamental discipline of traditional Chinese medicine (TCM) for at least 2500 years (VanderPloeg and Yi 2009). The earliest reference to the practice is in *The Yellow Emperor's Canon of Internal Medicine*, which dates back to the second or third century BC (Bowsher 1998). Traditional acupuncture has a unique pathophysiological concept of disease. It postulates the harmonious flowing of qi, a kind of energy, through a system of channels (meridians), as being the basis of good health (Kawakita and Okada 2014). Furlan *et al.* (2005) note that, in classical acupuncture theory, a sign of disease means that there is an internal imbalance between the yin and yang forces, which can result in an abnormal flow of qi within the body. The therapy focuses on restoring qi by manipulating these two forces, needling at different depths and at strategic points on the body. However, scientists still struggle to understand the concept of qi, since there is not enough anatomical and histological evidence to support its existence (Ahn *et al.* 2008).

Dry needling, also known as Western medical acupuncture, does not involve the concepts of qi, yin, yang or meridians, and claims to be a part of conventional medicine. Although the technique is an adaptation of traditional acupuncture, it has its own theoretical concepts, terminology, needling procedure and therapeutic application. White and the Editorial Board of Acupuncture in Medicine (2009) suggest that the practice is based on the current understanding of human anatomy, physiology and pathology, and the principles of evidence-based medicine. Western medical acupuncture lays emphasis on the concept of trigger points, and involves the insertion of dry needles into trigger points to produce a clinical effect. In addition, the therapy is primarily used to alleviate musculoskeletal pain, including myofascial pain syndromes (Cagnie *et al.* 2013).

However, the exact mechanism of action underlying the effects of both acupuncture and dry needling is still not fully clarified. Many hypotheses have been proposed to interpret the effects and mechanisms of acupuncture, but a unified theory based on scientific evidence is lacking. This chapter briefly summarizes pain physiology (pain pathways and modulation of pain perception), and describes the various theories of mechanism in the context of the evidence base for acupuncture.

Physiology of pain

Pain does not mediate through a single mode of action but involves multiple cellular mechanisms within the peripheral and central nervous systems. However, pain sensations usually associate two types of nociceptors (specialized peripheral sensory neurons): low threshold, that conducts action potential via myelinated A-delta fibres; and high threshold, that conducts impulses through unmyelinated C-fibres (Patel 2010). These nociceptive fibres terminate in the superficial dorsal horn of the spinal cord, where they form synapses via synaptic transmission. A-delta fibres form synapses in lamina V and I, and C-fibres connect with neurons in lamina II. A proportion of these neurons projects via nociceptive ascending pathways (spinothalamic and spinoparabrachial pathway) to the brainstem or to the thalamocortical system, where pain impulses are further processed and sent on to higher levels of the brain (Schaible 2007).

Modulation of pain

Peripheral pain

Peripheral sensitization of nociceptors (including A-delta fibres and C-fibres) is modulated by a variety of chemical mediators, such as prostaglandin, bradykinin, serotonin, substance P, potassium, histamine, interleukin-1 beta, calcitonin gene-related peptide (CGRP), nerve growth factor (NGF) and tumour necrosis factor (TNF). These sensitizing agents are usually released in response to cellular damage or noxious stimuli. In addition, local release of some of these mediators (e.g. substance P and histamine) causes vasodilation and swelling, which in turn promote the 'protective' mechanism of pain (Patel 2010).

Central pain

The modulation of pain does not involve only ascending transmission of impulses from the periphery to the cortex; it also involves descending control from certain brainstem areas (rostral medulla, periaqueductal grey matter), which regulate the ascension of nociceptive impulses to the brain (Ossipov 2012).

Segmental inhibition is an important mechanism that has been used to explain the modulation of pain perception. This mechanism is a subsequent modification of gate theory by Melzack and Wall (1967). The hypothesis proposes that the substantia gelatinosa (SG) layer that is located in the dorsal horn of the spinal cord is 'opened' by A-delta and C sensory fibres and 'closed' by A-beta fibres or by descending inhibition.

Endogenous opioids are involved in another mechanism that modulates pain perception via the descending inhibitory pathways. Three groups of opioid peptides (enkephalins, endorphins and dynorphins) bind to G protein-coupled receptors, mu-, delta- and kappa-, and are defined as the endogenous opioid system (Patel 2010). These endogenous compounds and their receptors are ubiquitously found in the areas of the nervous systems associated with nociception. The endogenous opioid system activates pain control circuits that descend from the brainstem to the spinal cord. The system is also able to provide analgesic effects by directly inhibiting the ascending transmission of impulses from the dorsal horn of the spinal cord (Millan 2002).

Besides the endogenous opioids, nerve activity in the descending pain control system can also control the ascension of nociceptive information to the brain. Serotonin (5-HT) and noradrenaline are the two main transmitters of this descending pathway. However, descending dopaminergic projections may also play a significant role in pain modulation (Benarroch 2008).

Chronic pain: central sensitization

In chronic pain conditions, the pain modulation balance is disrupted as a result of inflammation and nerve damage (Ossipov 2012). This altered balance influences neurons of the superficial, deep and ventral cord, causing significant changes in their response to pain inhibition and pain facilitation. This form of neuroplasticity, a so-called central sensitization, is often seen during cutaneous inflammation, or during inflammation in viscera, joint and muscle (Schaible 2007).

Central sensitization mechanisms are complex; it is hypothesized that different pain states might be involved with their specific mechanisms – at least in part (Nijs, Van Houdenhove and Oostendorp 2010). Central sensitization includes abnormal sensory processing in the nervous system (Staud *et al.* 2007), enhanced sensitivity of the spinal cord neurons, increased responses to stimuli, dysfunctional endogenous analgesia, lowering of threshold of nociceptive neurons, expansion of receptive field sizes, altered states of diffuse noxious inhibitory control (DNIC), and boosted activity of pain-facilitatory pathways (Meeus and Nijs 2007).

Mechanism of acupuncture in pain control

Since the use of acupuncture first sparked in the Western world, there has been a growing public interest about the therapy. Consequently, the need for scientific evidence for acupuncture's mechanism and effectiveness has become immense (Bowsher 1998). The scientific community has so far proposed multiple mechanisms for the physiological effects of acupuncture. However, most of these theories are heavily focused on neurophysiological effects. For this reason, this chapter will primarily concentrate on the proposed neurophysiological mechanisms of acupuncture for pain relief.

Neurophysiological mechanisms of acupuncture

Acupuncture needling has effects at multiple levels in the nervous system, including peripheral, segmental and central neural levels.

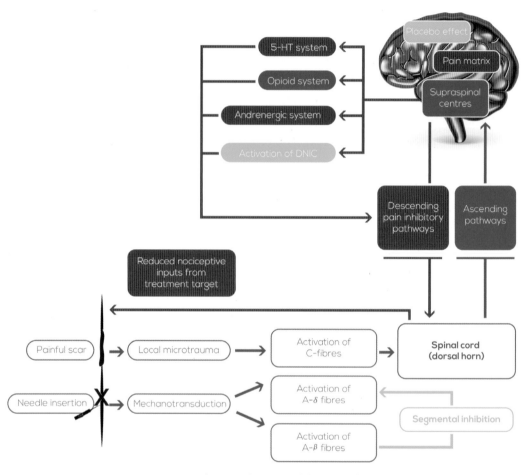

Figure 4.1 Schematic diagram of the physiological mechanisms of acupuncture-induced analgesia
Blue arrows = activation; red arrows = inhibition. 5-HT = 5-hydroxytryptamine; DNIC = diffuse noxious inhibitory control

Peripheral mechanisms

Acupuncture therapy has effects on local antidromic axon reflexes. Stimulation of needles in skin and muscle activates nociceptors, including A-beta fibres, A-delta fibres and C-fibres, which can induce an analgesic effect. Lundeberg (2013) suggests that antidromic stimulation results in release of neuropeptides from peripheral terminals, such as CGRP and vasoactive intestinal polypeptide (VIP), and other vasodilatory chemicals from the tissue around the insertion, including nitrous oxide (NO) and adenosine. These chemical mediators have either direct or indirect effects in modulating pain.

The release of CGRP has already been reported to induce skeletal muscle vasodilation in rats (Sato *et al.* 2000) and to increase blood flow (Sandberg, Lindberg and Gerdle 2004). NO helps to increase local circulation, which may contribute to pain relief (Tsuchiya *et al.* 2007). Adenosine has been reported to show anti-nociceptive properties during acupuncture in mice, though it requires adenosine A1 receptor expression (Hurt and Zylka 2012). Taken together, it can be said that local stimulation of needles may cause vasodilation in small vessels, improve nutritive blood flow and increase anti-nociceptive activity, factors that may be reduced in ischaemic and worsening pain conditions.

Segmental mechanisms

Acupuncture impulses ascend mainly via the spinal ventrolateral funiculus to the nervous system. To facilitate neural mechanisms within the spinal cord, acupuncture should be administered to tissues with innervation by the appropriate spinal cord level. Therefore, needles should be inserted into or close by the painful body part (Bradnam and Phty 2010).

Stimulation of muscles in the segmental acupuncture points mediates primary afferent nerve fibres (A-beta fibres, A-delta fibres and C-fibres), which terminate within the spinal cord (Pyne and Shenker 2008). These afferent nerve fibres form synapses with inhibitory interneurons within the dorsal horn, and influence three different sets of neurons: dorsal horn neurons, lateral spinal cord neurons and ventral horn alpha motoneurons. Acupuncture's influence on these spinal neurons is also known as segmental effects (Bradnam and Phty 2010).

Inhibition of nociceptive input

Stimulation of dorsal horn neurons facilitates the A-delta and A-beta fibre-mediated gate control mechanism, which results in inhibition of the nociceptive pathway at the dorsal horn by activating the descending pain inhibitory systems (Staud and Price 2006). In support of this theory, Cagnie *et al.* (2013), in their review, suggested that rapid stimulation of dry needles could activate both the large A-beta fibres and A-delta fibres, which could project afferent impulses through the dorsolateral tracts of the spinal cord to the central nervous system. This can more potently influence the supraspinal and brainstem areas associated with pain modulation. Furthermore, A-beta fibres have long been presumed to activate the gating mechanism (see

'Modulation of central pain', above); however, many studies have supported the hypothesis (Dickenson 2002).

In addition, Chu and Schwartz (2002) stated that, when a needle is speedily inserted into a trigger point, the local twitch responses induced result in a large afferent nerve fibre proprioceptive input into the spinal cord. This could have a central effect on the pain gate in the spinal cord, blocking the intra-dorsal horn passage of noxious information produced in the trigger point's nociceptors. Taken together, it can be said that activation of A-beta fibres can also project a segmental inhibition by interrupting A-delta fibres and C-fibres from forming synapses with the neural cells in the dorsal horn.

Alterations in sympathetic outflow

Neurons in the lateral spinal cord can alter the sympathetic outflow to tissues, as they contain the cell bodies of the autonomic nervous system efferent fibres. Stimulation of these neurons by segmental acupuncture at the appropriate spinal level has been presumed to produce strong analgesic effects by altering the sympathetic outflow to tissues. Lundeberg (2013) suggests that using segmental acupuncture points connected to a specific organ may alter its function by modulating both sympathetic and parasympathetic activity. However, effects on the sympathetic nervous system are intensity-dependent, and can be manipulated depending on the strength of needle stimulation. High-intensity needling increases sympathetic outflow and blood flow to target muscles, followed by a longer-term decrease in outflow (Noguchi *et al.* 1999). Low-intensity or non-painful input reduces sympathetic outflow from the segment (Sato, Sato and Schmidt 1997).

Changes in motor output

Activation of alpha motoneurons in the ventral horn by segmental acupuncture reduces reflex activity in muscles and enhances muscle relaxation (Yu, Wang and Wang 1995).

Segmental inhibition by acupuncture only occurs during needle stimulation. Since it mainly follows an opioidergic mechanism of action (Bowsher 1998), it may explain the short-term analgesic effect of acupuncture but cannot explain any prolonged or delayed pain relief.

Central mechanisms

Peripheral stimulation of acupuncture points mediates the mechanoreceptors, which send afferent signals through the spinothalamic pathway to the central nervous system (CNS). These ascending signals affect many brain areas (especially the hypothalamus) and activate the relevant brain nuclei that modulate analgesia (Cao 2002). On their way to the CNS, these nerve impulses project to the periaqueductal grey area and neurons in the rostroventral medulla. From there, they lead to the activation of descending pain inhibitory systems. This loop usually involves the release of endogenous opioid peptides (enkephalins and β-endorphins), monoamines (serotonin and noradrenaline) and GABA (γ-amino-butyric acid) and glycine (Lundeberg 2013). However, a number of other descending inhibitory pathways, originating at the brainstem level, may exist as well. The DNIC (diffuse noxious inhibitory control) system is one of them, which may be stimulated as a result of painful and intense needling (Leung 2012).

Endogenous opioid theory

The release of endogenous opioids has been the most well-known mechanism of acupuncture analgesia. The first proposal of an opioidergic mechanism was based on a groundbreaking finding that naloxone is able to block or reverse the analgesic effects of acupuncture (Pomeranz and Chiu 1976). However, the theory came to other researchers' attention when Fine, Milano and Hare (1988) reported that the pain relief activity of bupivacaine, a local anaesthetic drug of the amino amide group, was also reversed by naloxone. This new finding, in turn, provided strong evidence to support acupuncture's opioidergic mechanisms.

Since the proposal of the hypothesis, many studies have further supported opioidergic mechanisms of acupuncture. In addition, it is now disclosed that different kinds of endogenous opioid peptides, including β-endorphin, endomorphin, enkephalin and dynorphin, play key roles in acupuncture-induced analgesia (Chou, Kao and Lin 2012).

Serotonin (5-HT, 5-hydroxytryptamine) and noradrenaline have long been thought to play very important roles in acupuncture analgesia. It is hypothesized that stimulation of A-delta sensory fibres from needling may facilitate the serotonergic and noradrenergic systems. Chou *et al.* (2012) and Leung (2012), in their reviews, highlighted a number of studies that supported the theory for electroacupuncture to date. However, no specific experimental or clinical studies were found that support the proposed serotonergic and noradrenergic mechanisms for traditional acupuncture and dry needling (Cagnie *et al.* 2013).

Diffuse noxious inhibitory control theory

DNIC is the phenomenon where nociceptive inputs from sensory afferents are strongly blocked when a noxious stimulus affects the body, distant from their excitatory sympathetic fields. DNIC functions via opioidergic descending systems from the caudal medulla and requires activation of thin afferent fibres (A-delta fibres and C-fibres). These fibres travel down to all levels of the spinal cord to induce a potential inhibitory effect (Leung 2012).

DNIC system stimulation is another theory for acupuncture analgesia that is hypothesized to explain the immediate suppression of pain. The theory also proposes that DNIC may be the mechanism behind analgesic effects when needles of acupuncture are inserted at points distant from the actual pain source – extra-segmental needling (Pyne and Shenker 2008). In support of this theory, Bing, Villanueva and Bars (1991), based on studies in rat medulla, suggested that manual needling to the Zusanli (ST-36) could produce DNIC-like suppression and that the naloxone partially antagonized the pain relief effect. However, two clinical studies done on both healthy and whiplash patients have recently reported that DNIC on immediate summation of pressure pain did not show any noteworthy response to manual needling (Schliessbach *et al.* 2012; Tobbackx *et al.* 2012).

Mechanisms not yet known
Segmental dysfunction

Segmental dysfunction has been understood as mechanical problems of the components linked to the somatic system: skeletal, arthrodial and myofascial structures, and related vascular, lymphatic and neural elements. Proper functioning of each of these links is related to the normal motion of the entire spine.

Segmental dysfunction is not a disease or a pain syndrome; however, the majority of patients with the problem may complain of pain. Watkin (1999) suggests that segmental dysfunction is a problem in the function of a spinal segment, which may cause symptoms without necessarily being caused by physical pathology. The concept has been found useful for patients who complain of pain but have normal radiological and laboratory investigations.

The sympathetic nervous system (SNS) appears to strongly mediate the signs of segmental dysfunction. Since segmental acupuncture at the appropriate spinal level can influence the SNS, it has been presumed as a potential intervention to treat segmental dysfunction. In addition, as acupuncture lays emphasis on discovering and treating the symptomatic segmental spinal level, treating segmentally can be of diagnostic value in discovering the correct dysfunctional segment. However, there seems to have been no investigation on how acupuncture affects the measurable components of the dysfunctional segment. Therefore, it has been identified as a rich field for research (Watkin 1999).

Peripheral neuropathy (Gunn's theories)

Gunn (1989) proposed a peripheral neuropathy model to explain myofascial pain in a new way. This model suggests that, although pain may be linked to the signals of tissue injury, pain does not always signal injury, nor does injury always generate pain: pain perception can arise from non-noxious input. The model blames neuropathic pain on abnormal function in nerves. It also suggests that pain can become persistent due to ongoing nociception or inflammation, psychologic factors (such as a somatization disorder, depression or operant learning processes) and abnormal function in the nervous system.

Gunn defined peripheral neuropathy as a disease that results from disturbed or abnormal function in the peripheral nervous system with or without an altered structure. He suggested that a neuropathic nerve could deceptively appear normal: it might still conduct nerve impulses, synthesize and release transmitted substances and evoke action potentials and muscle contraction (Gunn 1990). In addition, Gunn (2003) also denoted the manifestations of neuropathy as radiculopathy (i.e. neuropathy at the nerve root), since they are usually found in both dorsal and ventral rami of the segmental nerve.

Gunn's model of neuropathic pain is founded upon Cannon and Rosenblueth's (1949, p.5) Law of Denervation, which states that 'when a unit is destroyed in a series of efferent neurons, an increased irritability to chemical agents develops in the isolated structure or structures, the effect being maximal in the part directly denervated'.

Based on this law, Gunn suggested that the goal in treating myofascial pain should be to desensitize super-sensitivity by restoring the flow of impulses in a peripheral nerve. But chronic myofascial pain does not usually occur without contractures and muscle shortening; therefore, their release was suggested to restore joint range and relieve pain. However, contracture-release requires a definitive procedure, such as physical stimulus, to decompress the nerve root and thereby break the vicious circle, as it does not release with conventional treatment.

Gunn claimed that accurate and repeated needling is the only effective way to release the contracture and disperse any dense, fibrotic tissue entrapping a nerve root. He introduced Intramuscular Stimulation (IMS), an alternative system of diagnosis and dry needling based on a radiculopathy model, for the management of chronic myofascial pain (Gunn 2003).

Clinical reasoning approach: the layering method

The layering method is a technique for acupuncture treatment to choose appropriate points and stimulation parameters in order to administer an optimum intervention. This method contains a series of questions that the clinicians ask themselves for clinical reasoning, so that they can evaluate the highly desired acupuncture effects for the patient (Bradnam and Phty 2010). Some of the common suggestions for the clinical reasoning questions include the following:

- If restoration of injured tissues or treatment of scar tissue is the main concern of the therapist, then eliciting local effects by acupuncture to encourage blood flow to tissues is useful. Local effects can be enhanced by using local acupuncture points, or simply by placing the needle directly into the injured tissue (Lundeberg 2013).

- If segmental effects are desired, then points chosen for local effects can be used, because these points can concurrently induce segmental effects. However, in the early stages of tissue damage when the rise in blood flow is significantly damaging, these points should be avoided.

Bradnam (2007) suggests that, in this case, any points that share an innervation via that spinal segment can be chosen (muscles, skin periosteum).

- If there is a slow-healing or chronic injury or a condition has a sympathetic component, then specific manipulation of the SNS can be used to alter sympathetic outflow to tissues (Bradnam 2003). Needling at the segmental points related to the target tissue, or needling a point in the periphery sharing the segment, can be used to stimulate the SNS (Bekkering and van Bussel 1998).

Are the therapeutic effects of acupuncture purely placebo analgesia?

In recent years, there have been many debates about whether the recorded physiological effects of acupuncture are purely placebo or more than a placebo. Opponents of needling therapies often argue that the mechanism behind acupuncture's success is nothing else but placebo effects, since studies suggest that expectations can actually modulate the perception of pain and involve subcortical and opioid-sensitive brain areas (Lyby, Aslaksen and Flaten 1999). They also add that placebo can activate the endogenous opioid system, as naloxone seems to reverse expectancy placebo (Amanzio and Benedetti 1999), like acupuncture-induced surges in pain threshold. However, a thorough observation of multiple studies suggests that acupuncture is more than a placebo and may have a more specific analgesic effect.

Acupuncture's delayed onset of action (by 1–2 hours) clearly shows that its therapeutic effects are not similar to the characteristics of placebo analgesia, which is typically immediate and short-lived (Price *et al.* 1984). In addition, once acupuncture therapy is ceased, its analgesic effects may last for up to 2–3 weeks, which is also very unusual for placebo (VanderPloeg and Yi 2009). Furthermore, several studies (Facco *et al.* 2008; Mayer, Price and Rafii 1977; White *et al.* 2007) have suggested significantly higher clinical effects of acupuncture compared with placebo.

Acupuncture-specific responses are also reported in neuroimaging studies. Multiple fMRI studies have suggested that stimulation of needles at Zusanli (ST-36), Yanlingquan (GB-34) or Hegu (LI-4) points may modulate CNS activities, including the activities of cerebral limbic or paralimbic and subcortical structures (Li *et al.* 2000; Wu *et al.* 1999; Yan *et al.* 2005).

Pariente *et al.* (2005), using PET scanning, found that the ipsilateral insula was activated to a greater extent during true acupuncture than during the placebo sham acupuncture. Taken together, these findings clearly suggest that real acupuncture is not just a placebo but has a more specific physiological effect. However, more work is needed to explain the definite neurophysiologic alterations from acupuncture needling.

Conclusion

After reviewing the current findings in scientific research, it can be concluded that the physiological mechanisms and effects of traditional and Western medical acupuncture are overly complex and involve peripheral, segmental and central neural networks. However, more insights into acupuncture's pathophysiological mechanisms are needed, since there are other mechanisms of acupuncture on the CNS which need to be fully explored. Studies researching acupuncture's neurophysiological and biomechanical mechanisms should, therefore, develop and apply adequate models of chronic pain to better explore the mechanisms. At the same time, clinical trials on acupuncture should have adequate sample sizes, use an effective needling technique, and have both a long-term and short-term follow-up to support its true clinical significance.

References

Ahn, A.C., Colbert, A.P., Anderson, B.J., *et al.* (2008) 'Electrical properties of acupuncture points and meridians: a systematic review.' *Bioelectromagnetics 29*, 4, 245–256.

Amanzio, M., and Benedetti, F. (1999) 'Neuropharmacological dissection of placebo analgesia: expectation-activated opioid systems versus conditioning-activated specific subsystems.' *J. Neurosci. 19*, 484–494.

Bekkering, R., and van Bussel, R. (1998) 'Segmental Acupuncture.' In J. Filshie and A. White (eds) *Medical Acupuncture: A Western Scientific Approach*. Edinburgh: Churchill Livingstone.

Benarroch, E.E. (2008) 'Descending monoaminergic pain modulation: bidirectional control and clinical relevance.' *Neurology 71*, 3, 217–221.

Bing, Z., Villanueva, L., and Bars, D. (1991) 'Acupuncture-evoked responses of subnucleus reticularis dorsalis neurons in the rat medulla.' *Neuroscience 44*, 693–703.

Bowsher, D. (1998) 'Mechanisms of Acupuncture.' In J. Filshie and A. White (eds) *Medical Acupuncture: A Western Scientific Approach*. Edinburgh: Churchill Livingstone.

Bradnam, L. (2003) 'A proposed clinical reasoning model for Western acupuncture.' *New Zealand Journal of Physiotherapy 31*, 1, 40–45.

Bradnam, L. (2007) 'A proposed clinical reasoning model for Western acupuncture.' *Journal of the Acupuncture Association of Chartered Physiotherapists*, January, 21–30.

Bradnam, L.V., and Phty, D. (2010) *Clinical Reasoning for Western Acupuncture: Acupuncture in Manual Therapy.* Edinburgh: Churchill Livingstone.

Cagnie, B., Dewitte, V., Barbe, T., Timmermans, F., Delrue, N., and Meeus, M. (2013) 'Physiologic effects of dry needling.' *Current Pain and Headache Reports 17*, 8, 1–8. Available at www.dryneedling.nl/media/Cagnie_jul29.pdf, accessed on 17 July 2015.

Cannon, W.B., and Rosenblueth, A. (1949) *The Supersensitivity of Denervated Structures: A Law of Denervation.* New York: Macmillan.

Cao, X. (2002) 'Scientific bases of acupuncture analgesia.' *Acupunct. Electrother. Res. 27*, 1–14.

Chou, L.W., Kao, M.J., and Lin, J.G. (2012) 'Probable mechanisms of needling therapies for myofascial pain control.' *Evidence-Based Complementary and Alternative Medicine 2012.* Available at www.hindawi.com/journals/ecam/2012/705327, accessed on 17 July 2015.

Chu, J., and Schwartz, I. (2002) 'The muscle twitch in myofascial pain relief: effects of acupuncture and other needling methods.' *Electromyogr. Clin. Neurophysiol. 42*, 5, 307–311.

Dickenson, A.H. (2002) 'Editorial I: Gate Control Theory of pain stands the test of time.' *British Journal of Anaesthesia 88*, 6, 755–757.

Facco, E., Liguori, A., Petti, F., *et al.* (2008) 'Traditional acupuncture in migraine: a controlled, randomized study.' *Headache: The Journal of Head and Face Pain 48*, 3, 398–407.

Fine, P.G., Milano, R., and Hare, B.D. (1988) 'The effects of trigger point injections are naloxone reversible.' *Pain 32*, 15–20.

Furlan, A.D., van Tulder, M.W., Cherkin, D.C., *et al.* (2005) 'Acupuncture and dry-needling for low back pain.' *Cochrane Database of Systematic Reviews 1*, CD001351.

Gunn, C.C. (1989) 'Neuropathic pain: a new theory for chronic pain of intrinsic origin.' *Acupunct. Med. 6*, 2, 50–53.

Gunn, C.C. (1990) 'Mechanical manifestations of neuropathic pain.' *Ann. Sports Med. 5*, 138–141.

Gunn, C.C. (2003) *Intramuscular Stimulation (IMS): The Technique.* Available at http://ubcgunnims.com/wp-content/uploads/2012/10/imspaper.pdf, accessed on 18 July 2015.

Hurt, J.K., and Zylka, M.J. (2012) 'PAPupuncture has localized and long-lasting antinociceptive effects in mouse models of acute and chronic pain.' *Molecular Pain 8*, 28.

Kawakita, K., and Okada, K. (2014) 'Acupuncture therapy: mechanism of action, efficacy, and safety: a potential intervention for psychogenic disorders?' *BioPsychoSocial Medicine 8*, 4.

Leung, L. (2012) 'Neurophysiological basis of acupuncture-induced analgesia – an updated review.' *J. Acupunct. Meridian Stud. 5*, 6, 261–270.

Li, W.C., Hung, D.L., Kalnin, A., Holodny, A., and Komisaruk, B. (2000) 'Brain activation of acupuncture induced analgesia.' *Neuroimage 11*, S701.

Lundeberg, T. (2013) 'Mechanisms of Acupuncture in Pain: A Physiological Perspective in a Clinical Context.' In H. Hong (ed.) *Acupuncture: Theories and Evidence.* Singapore: World Scientific. Available at http://media.axon.es/pdf/97162_1.pdf, accessed on 18 July 2015.

Lyby, P.S., Aslaksen, P.M., and Flaten, M.A. (1999) 'Variability in placebo analgesia and the role of fear of pain – an ERP study.' *Pain 152*, 10, 2405–2412.

Mayer, D.J., Price, D.D., and Rafii, A. (1977) 'Antagonism of acupuncture analgesia in man by the narcotic antagonist naloxone.' *Brain Research 121*, 2, 368–372.

Meeus, M., and Nijs, J. (2007) 'Central sensitization: a biopsychosocial explanation for chronic widespread pain in patients with fibromyalgia and chronic fatigue syndrome.' *Clinical Rheumatology 26*, 4, 465–473.

Melzack, R., and Wall, P.D. (1967) 'Pain mechanisms: a new theory.' *Survey of Anesthesiology 11*, 2, 89–90.

Millan, M.J. (2002) 'Descending control of pain.' *Progress in Neurobiology 66*, 6, 355–474.

Nijs, J., Van Houdenhove, B., and Oostendorp, R.A. (2010) 'Recognition of central sensitization in patients with musculoskeletal pain: application of pain neurophysiology in manual therapy practice.' *Manual Therapy 15*, 2, 135–141.

Noguchi, E., Ohsawa, H., Kobayashi, S., Shimura, M., Uchida, S., and Sato, Y. (1999) 'The effect of electro-acupuncture stimulation on the muscle blood flow of the hindlimb in anesthetized rats.' *Journal of the Autonomic Nervous System 75*, 2, 78–86.

Ossipov, M.H. (2012) 'The perception and endogenous modulation of pain.' *Scientifica 2012*. Available at www.hindawi.com/journals/scientifica/2012/561761, accessed on 18 July 2015.

Pariente, J., White, P., Frackowiak, R.S., and Lewith, G. (2005) 'Expectancy and belief modulate the neuronal substrates of pain treated by acupuncture.' *Neuroimage 25*, 4, 1161–1167.

Patel, N. (2010) 'Physiology of Pain.' In N. Patel and A. Kopf (eds) *Guide to Pain Management in Low-Resource Settings.* Washington, DC: International Association for the Study of Pain.

Pomeranz, B., and Chiu, D. (1976) 'Naloxone blockade of acupuncture analgesia: endorphin implicated.' *Life Sciences 19*, 11, 1757–1762.

Price, D.D., Rafii, A., Watkins, L.R., and Buckingham, B. (1984) 'A psychophysical analysis of acupuncture analgesia.' *Pain 19*, 27–42.

Pyne, D., and Shenker, N.G. (2008) 'Demystifying acupuncture.' *Rheumatology 47*, 8, 1132–1136.

Sandberg, M., Lindberg, L.G., and Gerdle, B. (2004) 'Peripheral effects of needle stimulation (acupuncture) on skin and muscle blood flow in fibromyalgia.' *European Journal of Pain 8*, 2, 163–171.

Sato, A., Sato, Y., and Schmidt, R.F. (1997) 'The impact of somatosensory input on autonomic functions.' *Rev. Physiol. Biochem. Pharmacol. 130*, 1–328.

Sato, A., Sato, Y., Shimura, M., and Uchida, S. (2000) 'Calcitonin gene-related peptide produces skeletal muscle vasodilation following antidromic stimulation of unmyelinated afferents in the dorsal root in rats.' *Neuroscience Letters 283*, 2, 137–140.

Schaible, H.G. (2007) 'Peripheral and Central Mechanisms of Pain Generation.' In C. Stein (ed.) *Analgesia: Handbook of Experimental Pharmacology 177.* Berlin and Heidelberg: Springer.

Schliessbach, J., van der Klift, E., Siegenthaler, A., *et al.* (2012) 'Does acupuncture needling induce analgesic effects comparable to diffuse noxious inhibitory controls?' *Evid. Based Complement. Alternat. Med. 2012*, 785613.

Staud, R., and Price, D.D. (2006) 'Mechanisms of acupuncture analgesia for clinical and experimental pain.' *Expert Rev. Neurother. 6*, 5, 661–667.

Staud, R., Craggs, J.G., Robinson, M.E., Perlstein, W.M., and Price, D.D. (2007) 'Brain activity related to temporal summation of C-fiber evoked pain.' *Pain 129*, 1, 130–142.

Tobbackx, Y., Meeus, M., Wauters, L., *et al.* (2012) 'Does acupuncture activate endogenous analgesia in chronic whiplash-associated disorders? A randomized crossover trial.' *Eur. J. Pain 2012*, 55. Available at www.dezuil.be/img/Tobbackxetal.EurJPain12.pdf, accessed on 20 July 2015.

Tsuchiya, M., Sato, E.F., Inoue, M., and Asada, A. (2007) 'Acupuncture enhances generation of nitric oxide and increases local circulation.' *Anesthesia & Analgesia 104*, 2, 301–307.

VanderPloeg, K., and Yi, X. (2009) 'Acupuncture in modern society.' *Journal of Acupuncture and Meridian Studies 2*, 1, 26–33.

Watkin, H. (1999) 'Segmental dysfunction.' *Acupunct. Med. 17*, 2, 118–123.

White, A., and the Editorial Board of Acupuncture in Medicine (2009) 'Western medical acupuncture: a definition.' *Acupunct. Med. 27*, 1, 33.

White, A., Foster, N.E., Cummings, M., and Barlas, P. (2007) 'Acupuncture treatment for chronic knee pain: a systematic review.' *Rheumatology 46*, 3, 384–390.

Wu, M.T., Hsieh, J.C., Xiong, J., Yang, C.F., Pan, H.B., Chen, Y.C.I., and Kwong, K.K. (1999) 'Central nervous pathway for acupuncture stimulation: localization of processing with functional MR imaging of the brain – preliminary experience 1.' *Radiology 212*, 1, 133–141.

Yan, B., Li, K., Xu, J., *et al.* (2005) 'Acupoint-specific fMRI patterns in human brain.' *Neuroscience Letters 383*, 3, 236–240.

Yu, Y.H., Wang, H.C., and Wang, Z.J. (1995) 'The effect of acupuncture on spinal motor neuron excitability in stroke patients.' *Zhonghua yi xue za zhi = Chinese Medical Journal; Free China Ed. 56*, 4, 258–263. Abstract available at http://europepmc.org/abstract/MED/8548668, accessed on 20 July 2015.

Chapter 5

Unifying Theories of Acupuncture

Fascia, Piezoelectricity and Embryology

Introduction

A unifying theory is a singular theory that can be used to define and explain all other theories. As multiple theories exist about the uses and different possible mechanisms to explain the action of acupuncture, this chapter addresses certain unifying theories, combining what is known about acupuncture and its underlying mechanisms as a complete and complex whole. A unifying theory is important because it gives a single theory to explain the diverse effects of acupuncture (from pain control to immunomodulation), which is currently lacking despite important advances, and aims to give an anatomical basis for the existence of the channels. Thus it attempts to combine these wide-ranging aspects into a single coherent synthesis.

In recent years, there has been increased debate among researchers about the mechanism of acupuncture in musculoskeletal pain and beyond. Since a number of clinical acupuncture studies have indicated a possible correlation between acupuncture channels and myofascial trains, and acupuncture points and fascial septa (Langevin and Yandow 2002), the possibility exists that there is an anatomical basis for the acupuncture channels. As research develops into the role of fascia, this may confirm or question certain principles of acupuncture practice (Finando and Finando 2011). Recent literature has described the concept of 'myofascial channels' as anatomical pathways that transmit strain and movement through the body's muscle and fascia. The strong correspondence of the distributions of the acupuncture and myofascial channels provides an independent, anatomic line of evidence that acupuncture's principal channels likely exist in the myofascial layer of the human body (Dorsher 2009). As a result of this and new and ongoing research, many experts now presume that acupuncture may work by transmitting signals via the fascia (McGechie 2010), a thin sheath of connective tissue that surrounds all of the body's muscles.

However, scientific evidence to support this claim is still limited, because medical literature rarely speaks of fascia in terms of its role in emphasizing the aetiology of acupuncture therapy. The rise in scientific papers on fascia and the new annual fascial conference is now bringing together a broad range of professions to foster understanding and collaboration among scientists working in fascia research and the various clinical professionals who address the fascia in their work with clients and patients. Part of this chapter is written to provide a basic understanding about the fascia and its role in human health and pathology, and to review whether there is evidence to support a relationship between the fascia and acupuncture. Also explored is the underlying mechanism of acupuncture, the development of the acupuncture points and channels and, in light of this, evidence and new research methods to evaluate acupuncture's holistic effects.

The acupuncture channel system

Modern medicine and scientific enquiry has always dismissed much of acupuncture theory due to the channel system having no anatomical basis, and has focused on the local effects of acupuncture. The channel network does not fit into the patterns of blood vessels, nerves, lymph ducts or any other known structures in human anatomy. As acupuncture essentially derives from channel theory, this must be kept in mind and investigated.

To date, among the scientific communities, there is no standard universal scientific validation of how acupuncture mechanics work as a whole to support the numerous studies and research projects that state the possible reasons for this mode of action. According to Tsuei (1996), this is due to the use of structures and concepts acceptable to the mainstream medical community with emphases on genetics, anatomy, physiology and biochemistry, and a near complete denial of energetic processes in the body (Windridge and Lansdown 2007).

Each of the 12 regular or principal channels is associated with a Chinese organ, such as the heart, pericardium, lung, spleen, liver and kidney (the yin organs), and stomach, gallbladder, large and small intestine, urinary bladder and tri-heater or triple burner (the yang organs). The Chinese organs do not represent the organs that share the same anatomical names in Western science and medicine. The principal channels are bilaterally symmetrical. There are also midline channels as well as connecting channels or channels that intersect the regular channel. Traditionally, the description of each of the 12 channels includes an internal pathway which 'belongs to' or 'permeates' its own organ and 'spirally wraps' its paired organ; and as such the channels spread on the surface of the whole body vertically and horizontally, integrating the inside with the outside of the body. The channels transform the whole body into one entire organ, providing the framework and unifying theory that all body functions are under the complete state of one organism and can be influenced by the channel system and corresponding acupuncture point (Wang *et al.* 2010).

Shaw and Aland (2014) draw attention to the fact that the words used in the *Nei Jing* to describe channels repeatedly contain the character for silk, 糸. They give further examples of where the character is further used: in the term for a channel network, jing luo 經絡, and in the term for an individual channel, jing mai 經脈. The conclusion they draw is that an obvious anatomical comparison is the fascia of the body which resembles silk in appearance. Reference to the fascia can be found in the centuries-old Oriental medical literature *The Yellow Emperor's Canon of Internal Medicine*, circa 200 BC. This classical text contains information that indicates that early physicians were locating the acupuncture channels within the fascia (Finando and Finando 2009). Matsumoto and Birch (1988) stated that such texts also described tissues and fasciae as important inner structures in human function. In addition, channels were given a plausible definition and purpose; acupuncture points were defined, and the concept of the circulation of an energy, or 'life force' (qi), via a system of channels, known as 'channel', had been developed (Birch and Felt 1999).

The channel theory was proposed based on empirical experience accrued over many decades and formed much of the basis of traditional Chinese medicine (TCM) (Finando and Finando 2014). The ancient Chinese were primarily concerned with the efficient manner in which acupuncture worked and developed many ways to promote stimulation of the channel system – from using moxibustion (heat) through to tui na (manual stimulation of acupuncture points such as acupressure) and movement-based practices such as tai chi and qi gong. The Chinese were less interested in acquiring a logical understanding of its mechanisms of acupuncture as we are in the West. Today there are many manual approaches to working with fascia.

One of the greatest problems of modern medicine is that Western medicine is fragmented into many different fields and specialities whilst acupuncture has just one unifying theory. The speculation is that fascia and connective tissue may be a key missing link needed to improve cross-system integration in both biomedical science and medicine (Langevin 2006).

With the channel system in mind, and the fact that TCM holds that individual points have specific effects, it must therefore be asked: what is special about the acupuncture points and channels and what distinguishes them from other neighbouring areas of the skin?

Holistic communication system

Myers (2009) considers the fascial web as one of only three holistic communication systems that would show the entire body if everything except one anatomical system could be 'disappeared' without the body collapsing. The three possible systems are the nervous system, the vascular system and the fascial system or web. (To find out more on this, go to Gunther Von Hagen's bodyworlds exhibition at www.bodyworlds.com/en.html, where he has done just that through a process known as Plastination.)

Myers proposes that there are only three possible holistic communication systems, these terms being defined as:

- *holistic* – emphasizing the importance of the whole and the interdependence of its parts and of or relating to the complete person, physically and psychologically

- *communication* – meaning the sending or receiving of information

- *system* – an interconnecting network; a complex whole.

When we think of body-wide communications, we usually think of the nervous and circulatory systems, as they support a variety of messaging functions, with signals carried by nerve impulses and hormones, respectively, whilst the third system is often overlooked.

The third system is the fascia system, often called the extracellular matrix, and is the only system that has direct contact with all of the parts of the body. While it is the fundamental material that our bodies are made of, the matrix system has not been recognized by Western biomedicine as an actual organ because it is so intertwined with physiological regulations and living structures that it is challenging to identify it as a discrete system (Oschman 2009).

In fact, the matrix is a dynamic and vibrant component of the organism, with vital roles in the moment-by-moment operations of virtually all physiological processes. Under the appropriate conditions, the matrix can react quickly as a unit. Signals can spread virtually instantly throughout the entire intermeshed system in an autocatalytic or chain-reaction manner.

Langevin and Yandow (2002) found that there was an 80 per cent correspondence between the sites of acupuncture points and the location of intermuscular or intramuscular connective tissue planes in post-mortem tissue sections. With such a high correspondence, they concluded that the anatomical relationship of acupuncture points and channels to connective tissue planes is relevant to acupuncture's mechanism of action and suggests a potentially important integrative role for interstitial connective tissue.

The connective tissue hypothesis: continuity and connectivity

Fascia refers to the soft tissue component of the connective tissue system that permeates the human body. It forms a continuous, three-dimensional and whole-body matrix of structural support, and is an interconnected network of fibrous collagenous tissues, which moves, connects and senses all of the body's vital organs, nerve fibres, blood vessels, muscles and bones (Findley and Schleip 2009). Findley and Schleip (2009) suggest that fascia includes aponeuroses, tendons, ligaments, joint capsules, retinacula, organ and vessel tunics, the epineurium, the meninges, the periosteum and all the endomysial and intermuscular fibres of the myofasciae.

Fascia's role in force transmission is well documented, with around 30 per cent of muscle force being transmitted to the connective tissue surrounding muscles, highlighting the role of the deep fasciae in the peripheral coordination of agonist, antagonist and synergic muscles (Carla *et al.* 2011).

Fascia is thought to provide ongoing physiological support for the body's metabolically active systems composed of specialized cells and tissues (McGechie 2010). In addition, LeMoon (2008) suggests that it keeps structural integrity, increases joint stability, provides support and protection, facilitates movements, contributes to haemodynamic and biochemical processes, protects against infection and helps in repairing tissue damage.

Classification of fascia

Based on the anatomical location, functions and distinct layers, fascia is classified into three categories: superficial fascia, deep (or muscle) fascia and visceral (or subserous) fascia. Langevin and Huijing (2009) coined specific descriptive terminology for different fascial tissues and provided details about each of these three categories:

1. *Superficial fascia* is comprised of the subcutaneous connective tissue containing elastin and collagen as well as some fat tissue. It is a web of collagen with a membranous appearance, appearing continuous and well organized to the naked eye. Microscopically, its physiological structure is better described as lamellar, resembling a tightly packed honeycomb. In addition, it is not present in the palms of the hand, the soles of the feet and in the face (Lancerotto *et al.* 2011).

2. *Deep fascia* is a layer of fibrous connective tissue that sheaths all muscles, and divides groups of muscles into compartments. It is devoid of fat tissues and forms sheaths for the nerves and blood vessels. It envelops all bones, including various organs and glands, and becomes specialized in muscles and nerves (Findley *et al.* 2012). The deep fascia is a highly vascular structure with superficial and deep layers, each with an independent, rich vascular network of capillaries, venules, arterioles and lymphatic channels.

3. *Visceral fascia* is a thin, fibrous membrane but composed mostly of reticular fibres. It encloses various organs and glands, and wraps muscle in layers of connective tissue membranes (Findley *et al.* 2012).

Classification of fascia is again reductionist to an extent because these fascial connections reach into the very interior of the cell. Findley (2011, p.3) describes this cellular connection in detail:

The living cell is a mechanical structure with a force balance between compression-bearing microtubules and tension-bearing bundles of actomyosin filaments. The tent pegs are the integrin receptors. The cells are anchored to the extracellular matrix by clusters of integrin receptors, which connect extracellular proteins and filaments to intracellular filaments, the actin-associated molecules. These integrin receptors also serve to sense physical forces outside the cell and transmit that information through mechanical connections throughout the cell to the nucleus, as well as to multiple locations in the cell. This cytoskeleton provides both mechanical structure and direction to biochemical reactions within the cell. The cell can thus convert external mechanical signals into internal biochemical reactions. In a similar fashion, development of the embryo is strongly influenced by the mechanical environment of the cell and is guided by this extra- and intracellular fascial network.

Schleip *et al.* (2012a) highlight the importance of fascia as a mediator of information and its role as a perceptual organ. The fascial network is our richest sensory organ. The fascial network has a greater surface area than any other tissue in the body, and the amount of fascial receptors may possibly be equal or even superior to that of the retina, so far considered as the richest sensory human organ!

Embedded within the fascia are many different types of sensory receptors, which provide important roles in proprioception, interoception and nociception. Proprioception is the ability to sense stimuli arising within the body regarding position, motion and equilibrium, and the fascial network is critical in this regard. Fascial tissues are important for our sense of proprioception, especially considering their vast distribution (Van der Wal 2012).

An exciting discovery of the fascial network is that many of the sensory receptors are interoceptors. The majority of these sensory neurons are so small that until recently little has been known about them. Interoception is thought to be a sense of the physiological condition of the body, provided in particular from visceral fascia. This subconscious signalling from free nerve endings in the body's viscera – as well as other tissues – informs the brain about the physiological state of the body and relates it to our need for maintaining homeostasis (Schleip *et al.* 2012b). Clearly the fascia is providing ongoing, complex feedback regarding homeostasis from a variety of sensory receptors.

Many receptors within the fascia are multimodal and respond to a variety of stimuli. The majority of these receptors are mechanoreceptors and therefore respond to mechanical tension and/or pressure. Of further interest is that certain types of mechanoreceptors (type III and type IV) have an autonomic function, so mechanical stimulation of their sensory endings results in changes in heart rate, blood pressure and respiration (Schleip 2003).

The fascia system is clearly intimately linked with the autonomic system, whilst the central nervous system receives its greatest amount of information from sensory nerves in our myofascial tissues (Schleip 2003). The stimulation of these rich and varied fascial receptors initiates a self-regulatory process.

The fascial system, like the channel system, can be viewed as one organ in which all organs and systems originally develop and which also has a homeostatic ability. The diverse range of conditions that acupuncture claims to treat may be explained by the recent advances in fascia research, although there is still much speculation (Schleip *et al.* 2012a).

Piezoelectricity

One of the most promising bridges for the correlation of Western medical science and TCM acupuncture has been in the field of bioelectromagnetism (Windridge and Lansdown 2007). Bioelectric phenomena are well known, and in the human body bioelectrical activity from the heart, brain and muscles can be recorded, displayed and measured. The theory is that the whole body is a dynamic electromagnetic balance. Cells and intracellular elements are capable of vibrating in a dynamic manner with complex harmonics, the frequency of which can now be measured and analysed in a quantitative manner by Fourier analysis (Oschman 2009).

Showing that connective tissue functions as a complex network would require evidence that a signal is generated by some component of connective tissue in response to a specific stimulus, and that the signal can propagate over some distance through the tissue (Longhurst 2010).

The piezoelectric effect is the property of some materials to convert mechanical energy to electrical current. *Piezo* is a Greek word that means 'to squeeze'. The effect was first discovered by Pierre Curie and Jacques Curie in 1880. Dr I. Yasuda in 1957 discovered the existence of a piezoelectric effect in bones.

Dr Julius Wolff in 1892 observed that bone is reshaped in response to the forces acting on it (not always beneficially, as in heel spurs, for example). This is known as Wolff's law. Mechanical stress on bone produces a piezoelectric effect. This effect, in turn, attracts bone-building cells (called osteoblasts) because of the formation of electrical dipoles. This subsequently deposits minerals – primarily calcium – on the stressed side of the bone.

An external electrical stimulation may lead to healing and repair in bone. In addition, the piezoelectric effect in bone may be used for bone remodelling. Wolff's law states that bone grows and remodels in response to the forces that are placed upon it. After injury to bone, placing specific stress in specific directions to the bone can help it remodel and become normal healthy bone again.

Clearly, mechanical stress is an important modulator of cell physiology, and there is significant evidence that physical factors may be used to improve or accelerate tissue regeneration and repair (Butler, Goldstein and Guilak 2009). Therefore there must be a feedback mechanism by which cells sense mechanical stress and thus remodel the ECM to meet those requirements.

Different biological tissues have the ability to convert mechanical and thermal stimuli into electric signals. Fascia in one tissue can convert mechanical stress into electrical signals. There is evidence that at least some of the channels represent low resistance pathways for the conduction of electricity; that stimulating a point on one channel may affect the electrical properties both on the same and on other channels; and that diseases and disorders can influence electrical properties at some points.

Over the last century, researchers have tried to scientifically identify these channels and acupoints on the body. In their experiments in the 1950s, Nakatani and Yamashita reported that different areas of the body can have abnormally higher or lower conductivity, and that such abnormal conduction is very closely related to the channel lines. These areas have been called 'Ryodoraku channels', meaning a good conduction line (Zhou and Benharash 2014).

Collagen fibres provide support and strength to, amongst other structures, bone, muscles, fascia, ligaments and tendons. They lie in long strands, providing conductivity to electrical charges that run throughout the body (Ho and Knight 1998). Therefore they have a dual function from cell to cell and tissue to tissue, offering mechanical support and a series of interconnecting wires that conduct electricity. Collagen fibres are often arranged in parallel, giving them high tensile strength and high crystallinity (sometimes described as liquid crystals) (Schleip *et al.* 2012a). When put under pressure or deformed, these fibres develop electric fields. Any movement gives rise to electric currents and fields, which is essential for normal cell regulation. Needling into connective tissue therefore may generate electric currents by means of mechanotransduction.

Langevin, Churchill and Cipolla (2001) suggest that deqi may be key in understanding how acupuncture transfers a mechanical signal into the underlying tissues. The hypothesis proposed is that needle grasp is due to mechanical coupling between the needle and connective tissue with winding of tissue around the needle during needle rotation, with any additional needle manipulation transmitting a mechanical signal to connective tissue cells via mechanotransduction. Further evidence in the field of mechanotransduction suggests that mechanical stimuli can lead to a wide variety of cellular and extracellular events and may in part be responsible for the various effects of acupuncture treatment.

The channel system is an early Chinese description of the now recognized fascial system. The fascia is an extremely good conductor and generator of electricity. Movement of the organs, bones, muscles, joints and ligaments all produce a piezoelectric effect at acupuncture points. Many acupuncture points such as the source points are found in highly movable areas of the body such as the wrists and feet (Yi and Encong 1996). The sensations felt by patients and practitioners of TCM during acupuncture, tai chi and martial arts were given names such as qi, and since these sensations appeared to move along the body, they were thought to represent a flow of energy. These sensations may well be piezoelectric currents flowing through the fascia. Acupuncture uses varied stimulation to generate piezoelectricity from lift and thrust techniques (amplitude) to rotation (frequency), whilst the size and diameter of the needle will also have implications.

Embryology, acupuncture points and acupuncture channels

It is widely believed that certain acupuncture points have different and unique therapeutic effects. Acupuncture is essentially a tool to stimulate homeostasis, and the choice of acupuncture points is therefore an important criterion because of these unique therapeutic effects (Zhou and Benharash 2014). Each acupuncture point has a unique therapeutic action (and often more than one), and a range of points is usually used for each condition.

Acupuncture points become tender or painful, because their sensory nerve receptors are pathologically sensitized. This is useful because it helps to determine point selection for stimulation and needling for the best clinical results. This sensitized condition is a dynamic process that is triggered by altered homeostasis, and returns to normal after homeostasis is regained post-treatment. Most acupoints show practically no sensitivity when the homeostasis is optimal, whereas they become tender under adverse conditions. Thus, the number of tender homeostatic acupoints may be a quantitative indicator of the health status of the body (Longhurst 2010).

Zhou and Benharash (2014) assert that trigger points share some, but not all, characteristics of acupoints, meaning that trigger points have some inclusive but not exclusive parameters of acupoints. It must be highlighted that acupoints share all the characteristics of trigger points, but all trigger points are not acupoints despite their high correspondence (around 70%, depending on source). Trigger points become activated through mechanical stress but are not pathophysiologically dynamic entities. A trigger point is classically defined as an exquisitely tender spot in the muscle, whereas an acupuncture point can be found anywhere in the body.

Nivoyet used sophisticated measurement devices, which showed that acupoints were about 50 per cent more conductive than surrounding points (Starwynn 2002).

In Western medical acupuncture the same acupuncture points are used as in traditional acupuncture, with many practitioners of Western medical acupuncture basing their choice on the same therapeutic effects but on the assumption that they are probably optimal for sensory stimulation of the nervous system (White 2009). If Western medicine is going to accept and use acupuncture more widely, it must establish the precise mechanisms of how acupuncture works and what acupuncture points are beyond the traditional metaphysical concept.

Shang (2009) draws our attention to the fact that modern biological models of acupuncture are inconclusive on a number of fronts. These are as follows:

1. The distribution of acupuncture points is different from the distribution of nerves, blood vessels, lymphatics or connective tissue.

2. The stimulation of acupuncture points has a multitude of varying effects. As a result this has meant that researching acupuncture's different effects has been complex and challenging, especially when you start to consider the number of acupuncture points and the number of point combinations as used in practice. Acupuncture does not have a single mode of action but a range of effects on various functions, whereas conventional nerve stimulation usually results in a unidirectional effect.

   For example, parasympathetic vagal stimulation slows down the heart rate and opioids inhibit gut motility. However, acupuncture at PC-6 accelerates bradycardia and decelerates tachycardia. Acupuncture at ST-36 suppresses hyperfunction (as in diarrhoea), and stimulates hypofunction (as in constipation), of the gut motility (Wong and Shen 2010). This suggests that some system other than the nervous system mediates the initial signal transduction in acupuncture treatment.

3. The therapeutic effect of acupuncture has been achieved by a variety of methods including needling, injection of non-specific chemicals, electricity, temperature variation, lasers and pressure. No conventional nerve stimulation technique has such diverse modalities of stimulation.

4. Acupuncture treatment is often very effective for a wide variety of disorders, with a long-lasting effect over weeks or months.

The growth control model

Shang (2009) proposed the growth control model as one possible explanation for acupuncture's diverse range of effects. This model can explain the functional, anatomical relationship and distribution of the channel system and acupuncture points. The growth control system is important in the formation, maintenance and regulation of all the physiological systems.

The growth control model claims that acupuncture points and channels are remnants of the growth control system, the first physical communication system in an embryo. This growth control system directs embryonic development, next to genetic imprinting. As every cell has its own place and function in the growing foetus, communication between cells is essential.

Cells start out with the potential to become anything, but early on during the course of development cells divide, migrate and specialize. In development, a group of cells called the inner cell mass forms. These cells are able to produce all the tissues of the body. Later in development, during gastrulation, the three germ layers form, and most cells become more restricted in the types of cells that they can produce. The cells are surrounded by a complex mixture of material that makes up the extracellular matrix (ECM). The ECM is a primitive fascia. This fascia is one part of the organizing factor of this development and proliferation of cells' communication.

As well as supporting cell motility in general, the ECM can confer direction on cell movement. In addition to acting as a guide for migration, the ECM can act as a barrier, ensuring that the correct structures develop in the right place. The matrix provides a three-dimensional space to guide their development. As well as controlling development by guiding cell migration, aggregation and the folding of tissues, the ECM can also control the process of cell differentiation itself (Davies 2001).

The extracellular matrix can be considered a structure to support and surround cells and regulate cell activity and is a lattice for cell movement. Functionally it provides mechanical support, embryonic development, pathways for cellular migration, wound healing and management of growth factors.

Cells can communicate with each other via gap junctions. Gap junctions are a specialized intercellular connection between cells. They directly connect the cytoplasm of two cells, which allows various molecules, ions and electrical impulses to directly pass through a regulated gate between cells. Keown (2014, p.77) describes the translation of the Chinese word for 'acupoint' to mean node or critical juncture.

During the multiplication of cells, communication between cells is impeded due to the increasing distance between them. When a critical distance is reached, two groups of cells are formed, which coordinate the cell growth around them. These groups are called organizing centres and determine the differentiation of other cells. These organizing centres are a small group of cells which control the fate of a larger region.

Organizing centres are characterized by more gap junctions, a lower resistance, a more superficial location on the embryo and a more negative charge compared with the other cells. Collagen fibres can transport impulses and form the communicating network between organizing centres, which is especially important when the distance is increased between them.

Acupuncture points and organizing centres are similar in several ways, including the presence of many gap junctions, a low resistance and a high conducting capacity. According to this theory, acupuncture points originated from organizing centres and are found on similar places on the body. Their network (connecting collagen fibres) is reflected in the channel system.

Based on the phase gradient model in developmental biology, many organizing centres are at the extreme points of curvature on the body surface, such as the locally most convex points or concave points which correspond to the distribution of acupuncture points across the body.

Shang (2009) described the growth control system as the foundation of pathophysiology. The growth control system precedes the development of other physiological systems and can be considered the template from which all other systems develop. As a result it is embedded in the activity of all systems, constantly interacting with them whilst providing ongoing regulation. Once growth is complete, these organizing centres maintain a level of regulation.

Shang (2009) considered that the acupuncture effect is a curious by-product of the growth control network. Organizing centres continue to function after embryogenesis. Stimulating acupuncture points or organizers can not only cause transient modulation of neurotransmission, but also alter the growth control signal transduction from regulation of various growth factors and growth control genes, leading to long-term effects.

Shang (2009) predicted that the growth control system had extensive growth control effects. Acupuncture has also been shown to regulate various growth factors and growth control genes, again demonstrating that acupuncture may work by stimulating the growth control network.

Many acupuncture points are located at transition points or boundaries between different body domains or muscles, coinciding with the fascial connective tissue planes. The growth control model suggests that channels originate from separatrices – boundaries in growth control – and form an interconnected cellular network that regulates growth and physiology (Shang 2009). These boundaries, as previously discussed, have high electrical conductivity. Organizing centres and acupuncture points lie along these boundaries; these are the acupuncture channels or channels found in the spaces between muscles.

Juyi and Li (2012, p.18) relate the growth control theory to early historic writing: 'According to the *Huang Di Nei Jing Ling Shu* (*Yellow Emperor's Inner Classic – Spiritual Pivot*), "The twelve channels lie in the spaces between muscles." Acupoints are the sites along these channels where one or more tissue structures intersect, divide or merge. These sites are referred to as "junctions" (节, jié).' These junctions are the organizing centres.

Acupuncture points have embryological relationships, which are clearly seen in clinical practice as treatment affects multiple systems simultaneously. For example, a point on the kidney channel may affect multiple organs along its pathway, including the adrenals, the kidneys, the uterus and testicles, because all of these organs develop from the same tissue when at the embryo stage.

The growth control model has also shed light on several puzzling phenomena of acupuncture, such as the distribution of auricular acupuncture points, the long-term effects of acupuncture and the effect of multimodal non-specific stimulation at acupuncture points.

Systems biology

Systems biology is one possible research tool to investigate acupuncture's mechanisms and effects. Systems biology is still in its infancy, but by using new mathematical approaches it has great potential. It is described by Harvard's Department of Systems Biology (2015) as:

> the study of systems of biological components, which may be molecules, cells, organisms or entire species. Living systems are dynamic and complex, and their behavior may be hard to predict from the properties of individual parts. To study them, we use quantitative measurements of the behavior of groups of interacting components, systematic measurement technologies such as genomics, bioinformatics and proteomics, and mathematical and computational models to describe and predict dynamical behavior. Systems problems are emerging as central to all areas of biology and medicine.

Yang *et al.* (2014) explain that the suffix '-omics' is added to the object of study or the level of biological process to form new terms to describe that information. This can include genomics from gene data, proteomics from protein data, and metabolomics from metabolic data. 'Omics' data helps to explore the different levels in systems biology from a holistic perspective, as it focuses on understanding functional activities from a systems-wide perspective.

Systems biology uses high-throughput screening, which allows a researcher to quickly conduct millions of chemical, genetic or pharmacological tests. The study can be performed on genomics, proteomics and metabolomics, and in the context of systems biology the tests have been able to identify potential candidates for the effects of acupuncture and provide valuable information towards understanding mechanisms of the therapy.

The principle of systems biology is to understand and compare physiology and disease, first from the level of molecular pathways and regulatory networks, then moving up through the cell, tissue and organ, and finally to whole-organism levels. It has the potential to provide new concepts to reveal unknown functions at all levels of the organism being studied (Lin *et al.* 2012).

Systems biology has created a shift in the Western research paradigm with a move away from reductionism. Reductionism is the belief that complex diseases can be understood by dissecting them into their individual subcomponents, and is no longer consistently the pre-eminent methodology of choice in biological research. Researchers are moving from reductionism to holism in their research approach and acknowledge the complex interactions between systems and networks as being essential (The Art and Science of Traditional Medicine 2014).

Other researchers have concluded that systems biology offers a holistic approach to medicine research and thinking and is vastly different from standard biological reductionism-based thinking. Chinese medicine can be thought of as a systems theory, and as systems biology becomes more accepted as a research method it will be valuable for evaluating the methodologies and outcomes of future acupuncture research conducted by Western standards.

There are many complications in studying acupuncture; for example, using acupoints on the lung channel could potentially have an impact on the respiratory system, the skin, nose, throat and large intestine, and therefore impact on a range of diseases associated with those systems. Reductionism might choose one aspect to focus on – blood flow locally at needle insertion, for example – whereas a systems approach would evaluate multiple aspects creating a more complex interaction. Again, acupuncture points and needle insertion have a range of effects, but these are situated in places that would not logically elicit these effects based on traditional anatomy. Lin *et al.* (2012), in their investigation of the use of systems biology to assess acupuncture, found that the acupuncture point Stomach 36 was the most widely used, having multiple therapeutic functions and targets, including spinal cord injury, allergic rhinitis, analgesia, neuropathic pain, anti-ageing, knee osteoarthritis and acute ischaemic stroke.

Systems biology is already being used by researchers to improve the delivery of cancer care and refine prognostic predictions for individual patients, as well as to understand the basic biology of the disease. Tumours are now being tested to explore each patient's unique genomic mutations. The same principle applies to complex diseases, which evolve from the interaction of multiple genes and environmental factors occurring at single points in time. But systems biology understands the body as a self-regulating, self-replicating system, constantly in exchange and dialogue with its environment. Each part exists in a delicate balance with every other part (Hill 2009).

Living systems are integrated wholes, and thus systems biology and research is now shifting from investigating the parts to the whole. The whole is more than the sum of its parts and, what is more, is about relationships. So systems thinking is thinking in terms of relationships, something TCM has being doing for thousands of years. TCM is a personal therapy that is holistic, with an emphasis on the complex interaction of the human body and the relationship between a human and its social and natural environment.

Sceptics of TCM could argue that using systems biology to explain acupuncture failure is yet another sophisticated way of stating why TCM doesn't fit into a standard double-blind clinical trial. However, it is now emerging that research and scientific evidence is finally accepting that living organisms are complex, non-linear dynamical systems by nature.

Systems biology is not without its problems, and designing clinical trials is problematic due to the huge range of parameters potentially involved and then understanding and interpreting the huge data sets generated. The hope is that disease-oriented studies using systems biology analyses will be able to capture the dynamics of change in molecular events, reflecting the beneficial change associated with acupuncture treatment, and become a preferred strategy for future acupuncture research.

Conclusion

The identification of the fascial system as a holistic communication system is an important one. It provides the framework for understanding intercommunication within a complex and living organism. Fascial tissue, because it is so intimately involved with the more specialized tissues of the body such as the organs, must naturally possess a broad ability to adapt physiologically. The fascial system obviously possesses a high degree of plasticity, and the stimulation of the acupuncture system may activate the self-organizing system of an organism and improve its structure and function at a more fundamental level than symptomatic relief. Acupoints are dynamic, living structures that change in the presence of pathology and dysfunction, and produce strong biological reactions when stimulated (Finando and Finando 2014).

Acupuncture is unique among fascial therapies because it employs various techniques to generate tissue stimulation and often does so at multiple sites simultaneously. It can be a robust form of treatment but can also be extremely gentle. Within a TCM framework it uses sophisticated patterns of disharmony to identify dysfunctions within a living system and in turn enables the selection of appropriate acupuncture points to promote homeostasis (Finando and Finando 2014).

The acupuncture channels of the East can be compared to the fascial planes of the West (Keown 2014), the phenomenon known as qi can be compared to piezoelectricity, and the dazzling array of acupuncture points and channels with multiple effects may be explained in part by growth control theory. Ultimately any disease will manifest in the tissues.

Whilst these theories remain speculative, they attempt to provide a unifying theory, although important aspects of TCM and acupuncture are yet to be determined. Systems biology takes a holistic approach to understanding TCM and acupuncture and offers a useful counterpoint to today's biological reductionism-based thinking.

References

Birch, S., and Felt, R.L. (1999) *Understanding Acupuncture.* Edinburgh: Churchill Livingstone.

Butler, D.L., Goldstein, S.A., and Guilak, F. (2009) *Functional Tissue Engineering: The Role of Biomechanics.* Ann Arbor 1001, 48109-0486. Available at http://people.duke. edu/~guilak/fte/FTEpaper.pdf, accessed on 20 July 2015.

Carla, S., Veronica, M., Andrea, P., Fabrice, D., and Raffaele, D. (2011) 'The fascia: the forgotten structure.' *Italian Journal of Anatomy and Embryology 116,* 3, 127–138.

Davies, J. (2001) *Extracellular Matrix.* Chichester, UK: Wiley Encyclopedia of Life Sciences. Available at http://onlinelibrary.wiley.com/doi/10.1038/npg.els.0001274/full, accessed on 20 July 2015.

Department of Systems Biology, Harvard Medical School (2015) Available at https://sysbio. med.harvard.edu, accessed on 20 July 2015.

Dorsher, P. (2009) 'Myofascial meridians as anatomical evidence of acupuncture channels.' *Medical Acupuncture 21,* 2.

Finando, S., and Finando, D. (2009) 'Fascia: The Mediating System of Acupuncture.' Workshop presented at the Second International Research Congress, Vrije Universiteit, Amsterdam.

Finando, S., and Finando, D. (2011) 'Fascia and the mechanism of acupuncture.' *Journal of Bodywork and Movement Therapies 15,* 168–176.

Finando, S., and Finando, D. (2014) 'An introduction to classical fascia acupuncture.' *Journal of Chinese Medicine 106,* 12–20.

Findley, T.W. (2011) 'Fascia research from a clinician/scientist's perspective.' *International Journal of Therapeutic Massage & Bodywork 4,* 4, 1–6.

Findley, T., and Schleip, R. (2009). 'Introduction.' In P.A. Huijing, P. Hollander, T.W. Findley and R. Schleip (eds) *Fascia Research II: Basic Science and Implications for Conventional and Complementary Health Care.* Munich: Urban and Fischer.

Findley, T., Chaudhry, H., Stecco, A., and Roman, M. (2012) 'Fascia research – a narrative review.' *Journal of Bodywork and Movement Therapies 16,* 1, 67–75.

Hill, S. (2009) 'Towards a systems view of medicine.' *European Journal of Oriental Medicine 6,* 2.

Ho, M.W., and Knight, D.P. (1998) 'The acupuncture system and the liquid crystalline collagen fibers of the connective tissues.' *American Journal of Chinese Medicine 26*, 251–263.

Juyi, W., and Li, M. (2012) 'The clinical significance of palpable channel changes.' *Journal of Chinese Medicine 99*, 5.

Keown, D. (2014) *The Spark in the Machine: How the Science of Acupuncture Explains the Mysteries of Western Medicine.* London: Singing Dragon.

Lancerotto, L., Stecco, C., Macchi, V., Porzionato, A., Stecco, A., and De Caro, R. (2011) 'Layers of the abdominal wall: anatomical investigation of subcutaneous tissue and superficial fascia.' *Surgical and Radiologic Anatomy 33*, 10, 835–842.

Langevin, H.M. (2006) 'Connective tissue: a body-wide signaling network?' *Med. Hypotheses 66*, 6, 1074–1077.

Langevin, H., and Huijing, P. (2009) 'Communicating about fascia: history, pitfalls, and recommendations.' International *Journal of Therapeutic Massage and Bodywork 2*, 4, 3–8.

Langevin, H.M., and Yandow, J.A. (2002) 'Relationship of acupuncture points and channels to connective tissue planes.' *Anat. Rec. 269*, 6, 257–265.

Langevin, H.M., Churchill, D., and Cipolla, M.J. (2001) 'Mechanical signaling through connective tissue: a mechanism for the therapeutic effect of acupuncture.' *The FASEB Journal 15*, 12, 2275–2282.

LeMoon, K. (2008) 'Terminology used in fascia research.' *Journal of Bodywork and Movement Therapies 12*, 3, 204–212.

Lin, L.-L., Wang, Y.-H., Lai, C.-Y., *et al.* (2012) 'Systems biology of meridians, acupoints, and Chinese herbs in disease.' *Evidence-Based Complementary and Alternative Medicine 2012*, 372670. Available at www.ncbi.nlm.nih.gov/pmc/articles/PMC3483864, accessed on 20 July 2015.

Longhurst, J. (2010) 'Defining channels: a modern basis of understanding.' *Journal of Acupuncture and Channel Studies 3*, 2, 67–74.

Matsumoto, K., and Birch, S. (1988) *Hara Diagnosis: Reflections on the Sea.* Brookline, MA: Paradigm Publications.

McGechie, D. (2010) 'The connective tissue hypothesis for acupuncture mechanisms.' *Journal of Chinese Medicine 93*, 14.

Myers, T. (2009) *Anatomy Trains: Myofascial Channels for Manual Therapists and Movement Therapists* (second edition). Edinburgh: Churchill Livingstone.

Oschman, J. (2009) 'Energy medicine charge transfer in the living matrix.' *Journal of Bodywork and Movement Therapies 13*, 215–228.

Schleip, R. (2003) 'Fascial plasticity – a new neurobiological explanation.' *Journal of Bodywork and Movement Therapies 7*, 1, 11–19 and *7*, 2, 104–116.

Schleip, R., Findley, T., Chaitow, L., and Huijing, P. (2012a) *The Tensional Network of the Human Body.* Edinburgh: Churchill Livingstone.

Schleip, R., Jager, H., and Klingler, W. (2012b) 'What is "fascia"? A review of different nomenclatures.' *Journal of Bodywork and Movement Therapies 16*, 496–502.

Shang, C. (2009) 'Prospective tests on biological models of acupuncture.' *Evidence-Based Complementary and Alternative Medicine 6*, 1, 31–39.

Shaw, V., and Aland, C. (2014) 'Channels under the skin.' *European Journal of Oriental Medicine 7*, 6.

Starwynn, D. (2002) *Microcurrent Electro-Acupuncture: Bio-Electric Principles, Evaluation and Treatment.* Phoenix, AZ: Desert Heart Press.

The Art and Science of Traditional Medicine (2014) 'Part 1: TCM today – a case for integration.' *Science 346*, 6216, 1569.

Tsuei, J. (1996) 'A Modern Interpretation of Acupuncture and the Meridian System.' 2nd International Conference on Bioelectromagnetism.

Van der Wal, J. (2012) 'The architecture of the connective tissue in the musculoskeletal system – an often overlooked functional parameter as to proprioception in the locomotor apparatus.' *International Journal of Therapeutic Massage & Bodywork 2*, 4, 9–23.

Wang, P., Sun, H., Lv, H., et al. (2010) 'Thyroxine and reserpine-induced changes in metabolic profiles of rat urine and the therapeutic effect of Liu Wei Di Huang Wan detected by UPLC-HDMS.' *J. Pharm. Biomed. Anal. 53*, 631–645.

White, A. (2009) 'Western medical acupuncture: a definition.' *Acupunct. Med. 27*, 1, 33–35.

Windridge, D., and Lansdown, H. (2007) 'Exploring the mechanisms of acupuncture.' *European Journal of Oriental Medicine 5*, 5.

Wong, M.-C., and Shen, H. (2010) 'Science-based mechanisms to explain the action of acupuncture.' *Journal of the Association of Traditional Chinese Medicine (UK) 17*, 2.

Yang, J.-W., Li, Q.-Q., Li, F., Fu, Q.-N., Zeng, X.-H., and Liu, C.-Z. (2014) 'The holistic effects of acupuncture treatment.' *Evidence-Based Complementary and Alternative Medicine 2014*, 739708.

Yi, X., and Encong, W. (1996) 'Acupuncture treatment and the piezoelectric effect.' *EJOM 2*, 1, 41–43.

Zhou, W., and Benharash, P. (2014) 'Effects and mechanisms of acupuncture based on the principle of channels.' *Journal of Acupuncture and Meridian Studies 7*, 4, 190–193.

Chapter 6

Current Research into Dry Needling

Acupuncture originated in the Far East approximately 2000 years ago, but only found its way into Western societies from the nineteenth century and particularly from the 1970s (Vickers and Zollman 1999). Within traditional Chinese medicine (TCM), acupuncture is based on the idea that the body has an energy force known as qi, which circulates around the body through channels called meridians. Health can only be assured when qi is flowing around the body with the right strength and flow. Acupuncture is applied to points along the meridian channels and is one way of altering the flow of qi. Western medicine has adopted the techniques of the Chinese method, but does not use its concepts. Rather, diagnosis is conventional (so a patient may be referred for back or neck pain) and treatment viewed in terms of conventional biology (Vickers and Zollman 1999). According to the British Medical Acupuncture Society, Western doctors trained within the Western scientific tradition do not accept the TCM understanding of the way the human body works. The concept of 'medical acupuncture' has been seemingly developed as a way to utilize the method for aspects of acupuncture that are viewed as having concrete scientific evidence for its effectiveness, and it is used alongside other forms of conventional medicine.

While there appears to be evidence that acupuncture works for conditions such as nausea and vomiting, neck pain, lower back pain, chronic tension headaches and migraines, amongst a range of other conditions, the National Institute for Health and Care Excellence (NICE) only recommends it for the treatment of lower back pain, tension headaches and migraine. However, NICE works within a framework of balancing clinical and cost effectiveness (Cookson, McDaid and Maynard 2001), so its rulings do not exclude findings of clinical effectiveness in other areas. The effectiveness of acupuncture is constantly being evidenced by medical trials, and advances made in trial techniques, so our understanding of it is not set in stone.

This chapter first discusses some of the contextual issues involved in evidencing the effectiveness of acupuncture, including the conceptual issues that arise when comparing the traditional Chinese approach and 'medical acupuncture'. It also discusses complications in medical trials, and how researchers have viewed these complications. The chapter then focuses on evidence surrounding the effectiveness of acupuncture on sources of pain. It explores the issue of the supposed equal effectiveness of acupuncture and sham treatments and the psychosocial issues that impact upon evidence, before moving on to outline evidence in relation to low back pain, neck pain, shoulder pain, knee osteoarthritis, migraines and chronic head pain, and cancer-related pain. An overall assessment of the effectiveness of acupuncture is discussed in the conclusion.

Acupuncture research problems

Research into acupuncture has had a number of limitations, including: incomplete understanding of the physiologic effects of acupuncture; the fact that acupuncture activates multiple physiological pathways, simultaneously achieving a local and whole body response; ineffective blinding of participants and investigator; unclear adequacy of acupuncture 'dose'; difficulty in identification of suitable sham or placebo treatments (sham treatments often have been criticized as being too similar to actual treatment); lack of clear difference between verum (traditional Chinese) and sham acupuncture treatments in clinical trials; the use of protocols and standardized treatment regimens rather than the individualized approach that characterizes most acupuncture practice; lack of standardization of treatment and selection of acupuncture points; inadequate sample size; inadequate treatment length; and biased interpretation of clinical results. These limitations make designing suitable methodologies difficult and must be overcome if acupuncture's effectiveness is to be evaluated. Nevertheless, despite these difficulties, there is evidence of the effectiveness of acupuncture.

Ahn and Kaptchuk (2005) encourage researchers to standardize treatments, as (1) the failure to do so creates uncertainty about whether we are studying acupuncture appropriately; (2) the variability in acupuncture styles creates ambiguity about whether we are studying the right style; and (3) the discrepancy between animal and human studies creates questions about whether we truly understand the underlying mechanism responsible for acupuncture's therapeutic effect. (Do animals and humans respond in the same way to acupuncture treatment?)

Langevin *et al.* (2011) argue that acupuncture needling has demonstrable physiological effects that are dependent on needling parameters – including needle insertion depth and type, and amplitude and frequency of needle stimulation – and there are different effects dependent on the needling of different body regions. Again, these effects may vary according to the precise needling location.

Langevin *et al.* (2011) recommend that acupuncture treatments should be studied both as 'top down' multi-component 'whole-system' interventions and as 'bottom up' mechanistic studies that focus on understanding how individual treatment components interact and translate into clinical and physiological outcomes, thus essentially focusing on both local and global effects. MacPherson *et al.* (2008) emphasize the need for whole-system strategies for developing the evidence without distorting the holistic practice of TCM, and encourage the use of qualitative research methods to explore acupuncture as a complex intervention. The use of qualitative research approaches also enables the exploration of some 'missing' topics in acupuncture research.

The STRICTA guidelines (Table 6.1) have been designed to improve the Standards for Reporting Interventions in Clinical Trials of Acupuncture. These guidelines provide authors with a way to structure their reports of interventions using a checklist. The aim is to facilitate transparency in published reports, enabling a better understanding and interpretation of results, aiding their critical appraisal, and providing detail that is necessary for replication.

Table 6.1 Checklist for items in STRICTA 2010

Item	Detail
1. Acupuncture rationale (Explanations and examples)	1a) Style of acupuncture (traditional Chinese medicine, Japanese, Korean, Western medical, Five Element, ear acupuncture, etc.)
	1b) Reasoning for treatment provided, based on historical context, literature sources and/or consensus methods, with references where appropriate
	1c) Extent to which treatment was varied
2. Details of needling (Explanations and examples)	2a) Number of needle insertions per subject per session (mean and range where relevant)
	2b) Names (or location if no standard name) of points used (uni/bilateral)
	2c) Depth of insertion, based on a specified unit of measurement, or on a particular tissue level
	2d) Response sought (e.g. deqi or muscle twitch response)
	2e) Needle stimulation (e.g. manual, electrical)
	2f) Needle retention time
	2g) Needle type (diameter, length and manufacturer or material)
3. Treatment regimen (Explanations and examples)	3a) Number of treatment sessions
	3b) Frequency and duration of treatment sessions
4. Other components of treatment (Explanations and examples)	4a) Details of other interventions administered to the acupuncture group (e.g. moxibustion, cupping, herbs, exercises, lifestyle advice)
	4b) Setting and context of treatment, including instructions to practitioners, and information and explanations to patients
5. Practitioner background (Explanations and examples)	5) Description of participating acupuncturists (qualification or professional affiliation, years in acupuncture practice, other relevant experience)
6. Control or comparator interventions (Explanations and examples)	6a) Rationale for the control or comparator in the context of the research question, with sources that justify this choice
	6b) Precise description of the control or comparator. If sham acupuncture or any other type of acupuncture-like control is used, provide details as for items 1 to 3 above

In order to distinguish medical approaches from the traditional Chinese approach, practitioners sometimes refer to what they do as 'dry needling' or 'medical acupuncture' – the insertion of a solid filament needle into trigger points. Claire Waumsley, of the Dry Needling Institute, argues that dry needling is different from traditional acupuncture. Traditional acupuncture is the 'diagnosis and treatment of pathological conditions including visceral and systemic dysfunction, while dry needling is used for the assessment and treatment of myofascial pain syndromes and dysfunction due to myofascial trigger points/tension areas/muscle spasm/increased tonicity' (Waumsley 2015, p.1). So in this respect acupuncture can only be used to describe the use of the meridian system, whereas dry needling uses the concept of trigger points. Trigger point dry needling is also used to describe the practice, but as with dry needling it focuses on the trigger point as a point of tension or tenderness – or elsewhere described as 'dry knots' (JOSPT 2013) – within the muscle that needs to be released. JOSPT (2013) and Kietrys *et al.* (2013) have suggested that it is an effective way of treating muscle pain; in particular, the insertion of a needle into the trigger point has been associated with a 'twitch', which may be a sign that the treatment is helpful.

However, according to the Wisconsin Society of Certified Acupuncturists, dry needling is in fact acupuncture, given that it involves the insertion of needles into the skin, and that the term is only used by those who have not been licensed by law (in the USA) to practise acupuncture (WISCA 2015). This would appear to be confirmed by Waumsley (2015), who argues that dry needling as a term is preferred by physiotherapists, osteopaths, chiropractors and manual therapists, because there is no need to train in traditional acupuncture methods. Meridian-based acupuncturists are dismissive of dry needling, with one referring to it as a 'crude and most elementary' form of acupuncture, which causes pain to patients and which is often practised after very little training (Meridian Acupuncture and Herbal Medicine 2012). However, Vickers and Zollman (1999, p.973) bypass such sectorial arguments by stating:

> It is often implied that a clear and firm distinction exists between traditional and Western acupuncture, but the two approaches overlap considerably. Moreover, traditional acupuncture is not a single, historically stable therapy. There are many different schools – for example, Japanese

practitioners differ from their Chinese counterparts by using mainly shallow needle insertion.

The impact of the various forms and techniques of acupuncture on medical trials

There are some difficulties in the literature with regard to terminology. While some medical trials impose a clear definition on the type of technique being tested, not all do (Foell 2013). Further, while medical science may be averse to using the terminology of traditional Chinese medicine, it is clear that some important trials have in fact tested this technique (Haake, Muller and Schade-Brittinger 2007). Johnson (2006) argues that the imprecise definition tends to bias conclusions towards a negligible effect. Given that traditional acupuncturists contend that dry needling is not 'real' acupuncture, the argument will be that only the meridian-based system can deliver real success. Further, many studies point to a range of innovations in acupuncture techniques (such as laser acupuncture), which complicates the assessment of the evidence (Johnson 2006). Finally, some trials are based upon the innovation of techniques by the acupuncturist to suit the particular condition to be treated (Blossfeldt 2004).

It should also be borne in mind that the scientific testing of acupuncture using randomly controlled trials (RCTs) uses what is referred to as 'sham' acupuncture as a 'control' or 'placebo' – this is where needles are used superficially on the skin (Hasegawa, Baptista and de Souza 2014). It is unclear whether this can offer a real placebo effect, because in some trials sham was found to be more effective than routine care, with similar effectiveness to acupuncture (Haake *et al.* 2007). This chapter discusses this phenomenon later. Further, there are different kinds of sham techniques – including partial needling, resting the needle on the skin and needling non-acupuncture points – making studies hard to compare (Hasegawa *et al.* 2014). While Madsen, Gøtzsche and Hróbjartsson (2009) conducted a systematic review and meta-analysis on the impact of different types of sham techniques and concluded that there were no *statistically significant* differences between different sham techniques, they nevertheless argue that further controls would be needed to make the placebo effect of sham more effective; for example, blinding acupuncture clinicians to the hypothesis of the trial, controlling the environment with regard to the site of needling, controlling the treatment ritual, and eliminating the effects of patient–provider interaction.

Complicating trials also is that not all subjects respond to acupuncture (Bowsher 1998), and some may be predisposed – whether by trait, context or expectations – to respond to placebos (Kong *et al.* 2013). Finally, it is difficult to control individual differences in the experience of pain (Lund and Lundeberg 2006). Johnson (2006) argues that there needs to be more consistency across medical trials in general in terms of the form and dose of acupuncture as well as controlling for other variables, although it was noted that there had been recent improvements.

In order to narrow down the focus of evidence, this chapter focuses on mainstream medical trials that involve acupuncture needles alone, whether this is referred to as the traditional Chinese approach or dry needling (and as has already been pointed out, it is often not clear which is being tested or whether the practitioner views them as being distinct techniques). Although much of the research generated through journals is extremely important, a reliable source of evidential assessment will always be the Cochrane reviews, which assess the reliability and validity of data alongside comparing findings from all available trials. In addition, as MacPherson and Hammerschlag (2012) have pointed out, the results of meta-analyses are also important, as they pool data sets rather than assess individual studies. However, there are also some key, and frequently cited, RCTs, such as Haake *et al.* (2007), which need to be included. It appears that there has been a genuine attempt by medical science to establish the effectiveness of acupuncture in treating a variety of conditions.

The section following focuses on the issue of pain and how to assess the effectiveness of acupuncture for pain relief, control and function. The chapter then summarizes evidence from systemic reviews and trials regarding low back pain, neck pain, shoulder pain, knee osteoarthritis, migraines and chronic head pain, and cancer-related pain.

Acupuncture for pain relief and control: the science and complications of effectiveness and efficacy

MacPherson and Hammerschlag (2012) argue that it is important to distinguish between effectiveness and efficacy when thinking about data relating to pain relief and control. Effectiveness concerns whether acupuncture has any impact beyond that of a placebo – that is, the outcome of the particular treatment is measured – while efficacy concerns the trial itself, and whether bias effects have been limited. They argue that studies have shown that acupuncture is effective for low back pain, migraine and headache, and osteoarthritis of the knee, and that the differences between acupuncture and non-acupuncture, while small, were clinically significant. With regard to efficacy, they also conclude that there are differences between real and sham acupuncture, albeit the differences are smaller than for effectiveness.

Acupuncture is viewed as a holistic, complementary and alternative medicine that stands outside of the Western scientific tradition. How it 'works' is generally not understood, but there are several theories and studies which have attempted to interrogate it via the terminology of medical science. According to Vickers and Zollman (1999), acupuncture can be partly explained through a physiological model.

Acupuncture is known to stimulate A-delta fibres entering the dorsal horn of the spinal cord. These mediate segmental inhibition of pain impulses carried in the slower, unmyelinated C-fibres and, through connections in the midbrain, enhance descending inhibition of C-fibre pain impulses at other levels of the spinal cord. This helps explain why acupuncture needles in one part of the body can affect pain sensation in another region. Acupuncture is also known to stimulate the release of endogenous opioids and other neurotransmitters such as serotonin. This is likely to be another mechanism for acupuncture's effects, such as in acute pain and in substance misuse (Vickers and Zollman 1999).

Bowsher (1998) points to various mechanisms of effect in acupuncture, including it being opioidergic, related to the positioning of nerve bundles and the operation of the sympathetic nervous system, and involving the release of serotonin.

MacPherson and Hammerschlag (2012) assess the evidence for the physiological underpinning of acupuncture and point to two general approaches to understanding its effects. The first involves the identification of biomarkers, such as 'antinociceptive endogenous opioids, immune system markers, cardiovascular activity, gastrointestinal function and fMRI-detected brain activity' (p.144). The second attempts to locate the effect of acupuncture within 'anatomical, biochemical and physiological bases of acupuncture phenomena, including those associated with acupuncture points and meridians' (p.144). These include a correlation between nerve bundles and many acupuncture points, a relationship between loose connective tissue planes and acupuncture points, and the mapping of meridian pathways onto the nervous system.

From the perspective of medical science, this has to be seen as speculation only, as it is generally agreed across the literature that the mechanism of acupuncture remains unknown. The unknown qualities of acupuncture are confirmed by Vickers and Zollman (1999, p.974), who say that some physiological findings of acupuncture 'resist conventional explanation'.

With regard to efficacy, in practically all of the medical trials this chapter has explored, there is a thorny issue of the near-equal effectiveness of real and sham acupuncture. Both Bowsher (1998) and MacPherson and Hammerschlag (2012) aim to show that acupuncture is an effective treatment regardless of issues of placebo. Yet the close correlation between the effectiveness of both acupuncture and sham is possibly an issue that should not be left 'hanging', with a minor statistical difference between the effectiveness of both being the point of dispute, because it is one of the main reasons medical science dismisses the potential of acupuncture. There are other ways of understanding how acupuncture may work and, indeed, provide a robust contribution to the treatment of pain.

One approach to exploring how acupuncture works and why there is a close relationship between real and sham acupuncture is through an understanding of the psychosocial – that is, the complex relationship between the physical, the psychological and the emotional – and in this, factors such as the value of the relationship between the practitioner and patient as a core aspect of healing or holding, one involving 'touch' and 'talk' (Foell 2013, p.311; Stomski, Mackintosh and Stanley 2014), and the expectations and the beliefs of the patient (Sherman 2014), are key. One example of how this issue is pressing can be found in the matter of comorbidities, where patients present with one or more (related) pathologies and multimorbidities, or where patients have multiple (separate) pathologies. Such patients are a challenge for highly specialized mainstream medicine, and Foell (2013) argues that acupuncture has an under-explored role here and has been excluded from systematic reviews on multi- and comorbidities. This is particularly the case with issues of chronic pain, which often defy compartmentalization or even a specifically traceable locale. In this case, argues Foell (2013, p.312), medicine has to ask the question as to what is the best approach to healing: 'Is it about acupuncture or acupuncturists, the method, the professional role or the practitioner?'

An important RCT in this respect is by Haake et al. (2007). This trial had a large sample – 1162 – of patients with chronic back pain, and it directly compared patient response to verum (traditional Chinese) acupuncture, sham acupuncture and conventional therapy. At six months, the response rate for verum acupuncture was 47.6 per cent, for sham it was 44.2 per cent, and for conventional therapy 27.4 per cent; the authors conclude that verum was not superior to sham acupuncture, although they were both superior to conventional treatment. Haake *et al.* have an interesting discussion about the results, where they argue that acupuncture has a specific effect on pain regardless of the particular mechanism used. This may be linked to the interaction of the process of accessing acupuncture with the psychosocial nature of pain, and chronic back pain in particular. For example, Koes, van Tulder and Thomas (2006) point to the importance of psychosocial factors in exacerbating back pain into a chronic condition, and Pinctus *et al.* (2002) concluded that distress, depression and somatization are factors associated with the increased risk of chronic back pain.

Studies by Kalauokalani, Cherkin and Sherman (2001), Linde, Witt and Streng (2007) and Myers *et al.* (2008) all concluded that patient expectations played a role in the effectiveness of acupuncture. However, a 638-person trial conducted by Sherman *et al.* (2010) found that belief in acupuncture did not automatically entail improved outcomes. They conclude that the relationship between expectations and outcomes is more complicated than has been suggested. Part of the problem of the original studies, they argue, is that there was no consistency in how expectations were measured, so they created a 26-item questionnaire to provide consistency of assessment (Sherman 2014).

Contrary to these perspectives, however, White (2009) argues that sham cannot be considered a true placebo. The difficulties of inventing a proper placebo for trials arose when the blunt, telescopic needle was developed and is often the main method used for medical trials:

> …this device, even though it amounts to no more than light touch, has significant effects on the pain matrix of the brain, and is far from inactive. (White 2009, p.26)

Looking at the psychosocial effects of acupuncture is not to suggest that its impact on pain and physical healing is negligible – many studies have proved that it is. As Johnson (2006) argues, there are at least as many that prove effectiveness as those that do not. It is possibly the case that medical science itself may be beginning to understand the complicated relationships and subjectivity involved in pain, healing and wellbeing that acupuncture may be in a position to answer or at least be evidenced against (Lund and Lundeberg 2006). It seems important therefore not to be defensive about so-called placebo effects but rather reflect understanding about the nature of pain, healing and acupuncture as a psychosocial healing technique.

Evidence for the effectiveness of acupuncture for specific forms of pain

We now consider medical evidence concerning the effectiveness of low back pain, neck pain, shoulder pain, knee osteoarthritis, migraines and chronic head pain, and cancer-related pain. There is a vast amount of research evidence available that has explored the effectiveness of acupuncture on pain. A search in the online Cochrane library reveals 1748 results, while on Medline a similar search will yield 5974 results, and clearly not all of these could be referenced. The research for this chapter therefore focused on some of the key studies and systemic reviews and took a 'data saturation' approach borrowed from qualitative research; that is, the end point of research is established when the same themes or authors are thrown up with increasing frequency in the course of conducting research, at which point the researcher may be said to have an overview of the field.

Low back pain

With regard to low back pain, acupuncture is generally found to be effective compared with routine care, and as such it has been approved by NICE as a treatment option on the NHS.

A Cochrane review of 35 randomized controlled trials involving 2861 patients (Furlan *et al.* 2005) on the effectiveness of acupuncture and dry needling (the review does not distinguish between the two) with respect to acute and chronic low back pain found that there was evidence to suggest that acupuncture was more effective for chronic low back pain than no treatment or sham treatment in the short term, but that it was not more effective than other complementary treatments. However, when added to other conventional therapies, it relieves pain and improves function better, albeit the effects are only small.

Contrary to Furlan *et al.* was a randomized study of 26 patients with chronic low back pain, who were allocated to two groups: one group treated with acupuncture and the other with anaesthetic injection. Acupuncture was found to be superior to both in short-term, cumulative and sustained effect (Inoue *et al.* 2009). The sample size was small, however, and the authors conclude that larger studies are needed. Witt *et al.* (2006b), who performed a large pragmatic (Acupuncture in Routine Case or ARC) trial of various forms of pain, with a cohort of 11,630, found that acupuncture delivered both medical and cost effectiveness. A Cochrane review of 26 RCTs involving 4093 women (Pennick and Liddle 2013) concluded that acupuncture was effective in reducing evening pelvic and lumbo-pelvic pain. Cheshire *et al.* (2013) conducted a study of 61 patients in the Beating Back Pain service, which combines acupuncture, self-management and information to patients. They found statistically significant improvements in pain, understanding of pain, quality of life, physical activity and relaxation. McKee *et al.* (2013) aimed to test the effectiveness of acupuncture in an urban primary care setting in the USA with ethnically and racially diverse, under-privileged, under- or uninsured patients. They found significant reductions in pain in over 30 per cent of subjects, with acupuncture being delivered by acupuncture trainees for reasons of cost. They conclude that it could act as a low-cost model to deliver pain relief in urban settings.

A systemic review of the efficacy of chronic low back pain by Trigkilidas (2010) identified four studies that met the criteria of eligibility of being concerned with chronic low back pain, conducting a RCT, and was based on comparisons between acupuncture and standard care. The first, by Cherkin *et al.* (2009), found that acupuncture treatment significantly improved function compared with standard care. However, there was little significant difference between 'real' and sham acupuncture, which raised questions for the researchers about acupuncture's mechanism of action. The second, by Haake *et al.* (2007), has been explored in the previous section. The third, by Thomas *et al.* (2006), was a pragmatic trial of acupuncture for chronic low back pain, which demonstrated both physical and cost effectiveness at 24 months; the effects of using additional acupuncture over routine GP care was weak at 12 months, however (also a contrary finding to Furlan *et al.*, who emphasize its effectiveness in the short term only). The fourth, by Brinkhaus *et al.* (2006), was a RCT comparing acupuncture, sham and no treatment. They found that there was a statistically significant difference between receiving acupuncture and no treatment, but that the difference between sham and real acupuncture was not statistically significant. Trigkilidas (2010) argues that, for studies 1, 2 and 4, patients were recruited by invitation or advertisement, which possibly meant they were predisposed to believe that acupuncture worked, thereby cancelling the placebo control of sham, although it may also indicate that 'acupuncture works in an unclear physiological process or that it simply has a strong psychological effect' (Trigkilidas 2010, p.598).

A patient data meta-analysis of 17,922 patients by Vickers *et al.* (2012) found that acupuncture is effective for chronic pain (in this case neck and back pain, osteoarthritis, chronic headache and shoulder pain) and that there were differences between real and sham acupuncture; however, those differences were modest. They conclude, in a similar vein to Trigkilidas, that 'factors in addition to the specific effects of needling are important contributors to the therapeutic effects of acupuncture' (Vickers *et al.* 2012, p.1444).

There have been fewer studies on acute non-specific low back pain (ANLBP). One such study (Hasegawa *et al.* 2014), however, performed a RCT on 80 men and women with ANLBP to assess the effectiveness of Yamamoto's new scalp acupuncture (YNSA) for this condition. It was found that there were differences between the real and sham groups, with those receiving real YNSA performing better in terms of pain relief and a decrease in anti-inflammatory intake. While the differences did not meet the criteria for clinical significance, the authors concluded that there is potential in this method and that further research is needed.

A different approach has been taken by one group of researchers (Stomski *et al.* 2014) to the evaluation of the effectiveness of acupuncture for chronic low back pain. Rather than the standard RCT, the researchers conducted a qualitative grounded theory study – in-depth interviews – exploring 11 patients' experience of receiving acupuncture for this condition and, particularly, what the impact was of the consultative process. The researchers attribute the success of acupuncture to the environment and the processes involved in acupuncture, particularly the trust-building between practitioner and patient, the feeling of control, confidence and security within that, and the treatment as a feeling of sanctuary. This correlates to other, more recent psychosocial studies on pain, explored earlier.

Summary of findings

For chronic low back pain, acupuncture has been found to be effective in both the short and long term in improving pain, function and quality of life, and can lead to reductions in the use of conventional drugs. There are differences between the actions of real and sham acupuncture. Acupuncture was also found to be cost effective. NICE has approved acupuncture for chronic low back pain.

Neck pain

A Cochrane review of neck pain involving 10 RCTs and 661 participants (Trinh *et al.* 2006) reported that, although findings were limited in their scope, acupuncture was reported by participants to offer moderately better pain relief in the short term. An ARC study on neck pain with 14,161 participants showed effectiveness for acupuncture (Witt *et al.* 2006a). Research on the long-term effectiveness of acupuncture on chronic neck pain was carried out by Blossfeldt (2004). In that study, 172 patients were selected over a six-year period, of which 19 patients dropped out for various reasons, and all had undergone conventional and alternative treatments for neck pain. Interestingly, those who had psychological or psychosocial problems were excluded from the study. The study was experimental, in so far as the acupuncturist used a range of different approaches, from meridian pathways to trigger points, until a selection of points were found that seemed most effective for this condition. Each treatment was customized, with a different depth of needling depending on the sensitivity of the patient. It was found that 68 per cent of patients gained 'significant benefit' (p.4) from acupuncture, and that 40 per cent of those experienced pain relief effects one year after treatment. Two other studies also confirm the effectiveness of acupuncture used in general practice for neck pain (Freedman 2002; Ross, White and Ernst 1999).

Summary of findings

Acupuncture has been found to be effective in treating neck pain in the short term. A study by Blossfeldt (2004) pointed to the importance of customizing treatment in relation to the needs and sensitivities of specific patients.

Shoulder pain

A Cochrane review and meta-analysis on shoulder pain (Green, Buchbinder and Hetrick 2005, p.11) suggested that there may be short-term gains in using acupuncture for shoulder pain; however, the evidence was considered insufficient 'due to the small number of clinical and methodologically diverse trials'. The authors called for more trials. Since the review, Vas *et al.*'s (2008) RCT trial of 425 participants found that manual acupuncture applied to a single point alongside physical therapy was effective. Molsberger *et al.* (2010) conducted a RCT on 424 participants and found that acupuncture was better than sham and conventional treatments for chronic shoulder pain; however, the reliability of the trial was partially compromised by a high dropout rate in the sham group.

Summary of findings

Acupuncture has been found to be effective for treating shoulder pain in some trials. It is generally agreed that more reliable trials are needed.

Knee osteoarthritis

Scharf *et al.* (2006) conducted a large RCT (1007 patients) comparing sham (off-point) acupuncture, real/Chinese acupuncture and physiotherapy/ NSAIDs. Success rates were assessed according to a 36 per cent improvement in the WOMAC (Western Ontario and McMaster Universities Osteoarthritis Index) score at 26 weeks. Success rates were 53.1 per cent for Chinese acupuncture, 51 per cent for sham and 29.1 per cent for conventional therapy. Both sham and acupuncture performed better than standard treatment, but there was no statistically significant difference between sham and Chinese acupuncture. Witt *et al.* (2005) conducted a RCT on 294 patients who were allocated to three groups, acupuncture, minimal acupuncture (sham) and a waiting list group, also against the WOMAC index. They concluded that after eight weeks of treatment acupuncture is more effective than sham or no treatment; however, the differences between sham and acupuncture at 52 weeks were no longer significant.

Manheimer, Linde and Lao (2007) conducted a review of nine RCTs on the effectiveness of acupuncture for knee osteoarthritis. Acupuncture performed better for pain relief and function compared with waiting list groups. However, the differences between sham and acupuncture were not viewed as clinically significant. Manheimer *et al.* (2010) also conducted a Cochrane review of 16 RCTs and concluded that acupuncture showed statistically significant improvements in pain and function compared with sham; however, they argued that acupuncture did not meet the guidelines for 'clinical relevance'. Contrary to these findings, White *et al.* (2006) conducted a meta-analysis on five high-quality trials and found significant differences between acupuncture and sham, with the former being more effective in short-term pain.

Foster *et al.* (2007) conducted a multicentre RCT, involving 352 patients aged over 50 with a diagnosis of knee osteoarthritis, on the effectiveness of acupuncture on knee pain in conjunction with advice and exercise-based physiotherapy. They found small benefits in pain intensity and unpleasantness for the acupuncture groups, but that this was more sustained in the sham group. They conclude that the effects had little to do with acupuncture. The study, however, only used six sessions of acupuncture, which the authors argue may have been suboptimal.

In contrast, a longer-term (two-year) study of – initially 90 – patients with knee osteoarthritis (White *et al.* 2012) concluded that acupuncture showed effectiveness, improvement in function and reduction in stiffness according to Measure Yourself Medical Outcome Profile (MYMOP) scores conducted over the two-year period. The authors argue that using acupuncture as a possible alternative to knee surgery could save £100,000 a year.

Summary of findings

Some studies have found acupuncture very effective for treating knee osteoarthritis (reductions in pain and stiffness and improvement in function), while others have found similar effectiveness between real and sham acupuncture, or have found differences between real and sham acupuncture to be statistically but not clinically significant.

Migraines and chronic head pain

A Cochrane review on idiopathic headache (Melchart *et al.* 2001) examined 26 trials (1151 patients), 16 of which were concerned with migraine and tension-type headaches (TTH). In eight of the trials, real acupuncture was significantly superior to sham, in four there were moderate differences, and in two acupuncture and sham performed in similar ways. They conclude that there was some evidence to suggest the effectiveness of acupuncture for idiopathic headache but that there needed to be better-quality evidence to assess this fully.

Some trials since this review were less positive in terms of effectiveness. Linde, Streng and Jürgens (2005) and Melchart *et al.* (2005) found that responder rates were good for both acupuncture and sham (control) groups for migraine and TTH, and Diener, Kronfeld and Boewing (2006) found no difference in outcomes between acupuncture, sham and standard therapy for migraine.

New Cochrane reviews split trials between migraine and TTH. For migraine, new trials showed that prophylactic acupuncture was at least as effective as conventional drug treatments, with fewer side effects, although differences between acupuncture and sham were difficult to interpret or prove (Linde, Allais and Brinkhaus 2009a). Another Cochrane review concluded with new evidence that acupuncture could be useful for TTH (Linde, Allais and Brinkhaus 2009b). NICE guidelines recommend acupuncture as a treatment for migraine and TTH.

Summary of findings

Acupuncture has in most trials been viewed as effective for migraine and TTH compared with conventional treatments, with fewer side effects. NICE guidelines have approved acupuncture for both of these conditions.

Relief of pain in cancer patients

There are two sources of pain relating to cancer: one from the tumour and another from the effects of treatment. A Cochrane review (Paley *et al.* 2012) attempted to review evidence of the effectiveness of acupuncture for cancer pain, but identified only one study of sufficient quality (see Alimi *et al.* 2003). The review concluded that more research was needed.

Choi *et al.* (2012) conducted a systemic review of 15 trials (1157 patients) and concluded that, while the quality of the trials was not good, acupuncture could be more effective in providing pain control when combined with drug therapy than drug therapy alone.

Weidong and Rosenthal (2013) conducted a review of trials relating to acupuncture and cancer pain, and concluded that there was some evidence to suggest that acupuncture could help cancer-related pain. However, treatment needed to be combined with an understanding of oncology and in particular the progression of cancer in each individual patient. This again points to the specificity of the patient/practitioner relationship understood through the lens of medical science, in this case oncology.

Summary of findings

Recent research has suggested that acupuncture can assist with cancer-related pain. Weidong and Rosenthal (2013) suggest that a patient-centred approach is most effective – that is, when knowledge of oncology and the patient's specific progress was part of the treatment.

Conclusion

RCTs, pragmatic trials, systemic reviews, meta-analyses and other research studies tend toward agreement that acupuncture has an impact, particularly on chronic low back pain. Similar, yet perhaps less systematic, results have been found with neck and shoulder pain, knee osteoarthritis, migraine and TTH, and cancer pain. They further agree that there is a difference between real and sham acupuncture, albeit there is some dispute as to the extent of those differences and their statistical and clinical significance. Finally, the importance of the psychosocial effects of acupuncture has been noted in clinical trials, and there are differences in the degree to which this is viewed as discrediting acupuncture. Arguably there are lessons to be learnt from acupuncture in this respect, particularly in relation to the interpersonal nature of healing and what impact this might have on our understanding of training (what qualities make for a 'good' healer, and what practices are involved in healing).

Studies have also shown the cost effectiveness of acupuncture compared with conventional treatment, and this has relevance to situations of constrained resources. Put simply, if patients feel that acupuncture works and that this has a positive impact on their actual wellbeing, and that the method in question is cost effective, then it can be seen to 'work' irrespective of the findings of mainstream clinical trials.

However, it is not possible to say that trials have any degree of consistency across several variables, including type of acupuncture, extent of treatment and the type of sham or placebo used (Johnson 2006). Furthermore, medical science tends to struggle with psychosocial questions and the possibility of systemic treatments for co- and multimorbidities (Foell 2013). Many of the studies have concluded that better consistency of approach in RCTs, and more research, is needed to test the effectiveness of acupuncture. Increasingly there is perceived to be a need to understand better the mechanism of acupuncture, to explore the psychosocial nature of pain and the impact acupuncture has on it, and to reflect on the best approach to assess evidence as to its effectiveness.

References

Ahn, A.C., and Kaptchuk, T.J. (2005) 'Advancing acupuncture research.' *Altern. Ther. Health Med. 11*, 3, 40–45.

Alimi, D., Rubino, C., Pichard-Leandri, E., Fermand-Brule, S., Dubreuil-Lemaire, M.L., and Hill, C. (2003) 'Analgesic effect of auricular acupuncture for cancer pain: a randomized, blinded, controlled trial.' *J. Clin. Oncol. 21*, 22, 4120–4126.

Blossfeldt, P. (2004) 'Acupuncture for chronic neck pain – a cohort study in an NHS pain clinic.' *Acupuncture in Medicine 22*, 3, 146–151.

Bowsher, D. (1998) 'Mechanisms of Acupuncture.' In J. Filshie and A. White (eds) *Medical Acupuncture – A Western Scientific Approach* (first edition). Edinburgh: Churchill Livingstone.

Brinkhaus, B., Witt, C.M., Jena, S., Linde, K., Streng, A., and Wagenpfeil, S. (2006) 'Acupuncture in patients with chronic low back pain: a randomized controlled trial.' *Arch. Intern. Med. 166*, 450–457.

Cherkin, D.C., Sherman, K.J., Avins, A.L., Erro, J.H., Ichikawa, L., and Barlow, W.E. (2009) 'A randomized trial comparing acupuncture, simulated acupuncture, and usual care for chronic low back pain.' *Arch. Intern. Med. 169*, 858–866.

Cheshire, A., Polley, M., Peters, D., and Ridge, D. (2013) 'Patient outcomes and experiences of an acupuncture and self-care service for persistent low back pain in the NHS: a mixed methods approach.' *BMC Complementary and Alternative Medicine 13*, 300.

Choi, T.Y., Lee, M.S., Kim, T.H., Zaslawski, C., and Ernst, E. (2012) 'Acupuncture for the treatment of cancer pain: a systematic review of randomized clinical trials.' *Support Care Cancer 20*, 6, 1147–1158.

Cookson, R., McDaid, D., and Maynard, A. (2001) 'Wrong SIGN, NICE mess: is national guidance distorting allocation of resources?' *BMJ 323*, 7315, 743–745.

Diener, H.C., Kronfeld, K., and Boewing, G. (2006) 'Efficacy of acupuncture for the prophylaxis of migraine: a multicentre randomized controlled clinical trial.' *Lancet Neurol. 5*, 310–316.

Foell, J. (2013) 'Conventional and complementary approaches to chronic widespread pain and its comorbidities.' *Acupunct. Med. 31*, 309–314.

Foster, N.E., Thomas, E., Barlas, P., *et al.* (2007) 'Acupuncture as an adjunct to exercise based physiotherapy for osteoarthritis of the knee: randomized controlled trial.' *BMJ 335*, 7617, 436.

Freedman, J. (2002) 'An audit of 500 acupuncture patients in general practice.' *Acupunct. Med. 20*, 1, 30–34.

Furlan, A.D., van Tulder, M.W., Cherkin, D., *et al.* (2005) 'Acupuncture and dry-needling for low back pain.' *Cochrane Database of Systematic Reviews 1*, CD001351.

Green, S., Buchbinder, R., and Hetrick, S. (2005) 'Acupuncture for shoulder pain.' *Cochrane Database of Systematic Reviews 2*, CD005319.

Haake, M., Muller, H.H., and Schade-Brittinger, C. (2007) 'German Acupuncture Trials (GERAC) for chronic low back pain: randomized, multicenter, blinded, parallel-group trial with 3 groups.' *Arch. Intern. Med. 167*, 1892–1898.

Hasegawa, T.M., Baptista, A.S., and de Souza, M.C. (2014) 'Acupuncture for acute non-specific low back pain: a randomized, controlled, double-blind, placebo trial.' *Acupunct. Med. 32*, 109–115.

Inoue, M., Hojo, T., Nakajima, M., Kitakoji, H., and Itoi, M. (2009) 'Comparison of the effectiveness of acupuncture treatment and local anaesthetic injection for low back pain: a randomized controlled clinical trial.' *Acupunct. Med. 27*, 174–177.

Johnson, M.I. (2006) 'The clinical effectiveness of acupuncture for pain relief – you can be certain of uncertainty.' *Acupunct. Med. 24*, 2, 71–79.

JOSPT (2013) 'Perspectives for patients. Painful and tender muscles: dry needling can reduce myofascial pain related to trigger points muscles.' *J. Orthop. Sports Phys. Ther. 43*, 9, 635.

Kalauokalani, D., Cherkin, D.C., and Sherman, K.J. (2001) 'Lessons from a trial of acupuncture and massage for low back pain: patient expectations and treatment effects.' *Spine 26*, 1418–1424.

Kietrys, D.M., Palombaro, K.M., Azzaretto, E., *et al.* (2013) 'Effectiveness of dry needling for upper-quarter myofascial pain: a systematic review and meta-analysis.' *J. Orthop. Sports Phys. Ther. 43*, 9, 620–634.

Koes, B.W., van Tulder, M.W., and Thomas, S. (2006) 'Diagnosis and treatment of low back pain.' *BMJ 2006*, 332.

Kong, J., Spaeth, R., Cook, A., et al. (2013) 'Are all placebo effects equal? Placebo pills, sham acupuncture, cue conditioning and their association.' *PLoS One 8*, 7, e67485.

Langevin, H.M., Wayne, P.M., MacPherson, H., *et al.* (2011) 'Paradoxes in acupuncture research: strategies for moving forward.' *Evidence-Based Complementary and Alternative Medicine: eCAM 2011*, 180805.

Linde, K., Allais, G., and Brinkhaus, B. (2009a) 'Acupuncture for migraine prophylaxis.' *Cochrane Database of Systematic Reviews 1*, CD001218.

Linde, K., Allais, G., and Brinkhaus, B. (2009b) 'Acupuncture for tension-type headache.' *Cochrane Database of Systematic Reviews 1*, CD007587.

Linde, K., Streng, A., and Jürgens, S. (2005) 'Acupuncture for patients with migraine: a randomized controlled trial.' *JAMA 293*, 2118–2125.

Linde, K., Witt, C.M., and Streng, A. (2007) 'The impact of patient expectations on outcomes in four randomized controlled trials of acupuncture in patients with chronic pain.' *Pain 128*, 264–271.

Lund, I., and Lundeberg, T. (2006) 'Aspects of pain, its assessment and evaluation from an acupuncture perspective.' *Acupunct. Med. 24*, 3, 109–117.

MacPherson, H., and Hammerschlag, R. (2012) 'Acupuncture and the emerging evidence base: contrived controversy and rational debate.' *J. Acupunct. Meridian Stud. 5*, 4, 141–147.

MacPherson, H., Nahin, R., Paterson, C., Cassidy, C., Lewith, G., and Hammerschlag, R. (2008) 'Developments in acupuncture research: big-picture perspectives from the leading edge.' *The Journal of Alternative and Complementary Medicine 14*, 7, 883–887.

Madsen, N.V., Gøtzsche, P.C., and Hróbjartsson, A. (2009) 'Acupuncture treatment for pain: systematic review of randomized clinical trials with acupuncture, placebo acupuncture, and no acupuncture groups.' *BMJ 338*, a3115.

Manheimer, E., Cheng, K., Linde, K., *et al.* (2010) 'Acupuncture for peripheral joint osteoarthritis.' *Cochrane Database of Systematic Reviews 1*, CD001977.

Manheimer, E., Linde, K., and Lao, L. (2007) 'Meta-analysis: acupuncture for osteoarthritis of the knee.' *Annals of Internal Medicine 146*, 868–877.

McKee, M.D., Kligler, B., Fletcher, J., Biryukov, F., Casalaina, W., Anderson, B., and Blank, A. (2013) 'Outcomes of acupuncture for chronic pain in urban primary care.' *The Journal of the American Board of Family Medicine 26*, 6, 692–700.

Melchart, D., Linde, K., Fischer, P., *et al.* (2001) 'Acupuncture for idiopathic headache.' *Cochrane Database of Systematic Reviews 1*, CD001218.

Melchart, D., Streng, A., Hoppe, A., *et al.* (2005) 'Acupuncture in patients with tension-type headache: randomised controlled trial.' *BMJ 331*, 376–382.

Meridian Acupuncture and Herbal Medicine (2012) *Acupuncture vs. Dry Needling.* Available at http://meridianlouisville.blogspot.co.uk/2012/11/acupuncture-vs-dry-needling.html, accessed on 21 July 2015.

Molsberger, A.F., Schneider, T., Gotthardt, H., *et al.* (2010) 'German Randomized Acupuncture Trial for Chronic Shoulder Pain (GRASP) – a pragmatic, controlled, patient-blinded, multi-centre trial in an outpatient care environment.' *Pain 151*, 146–154.

Myers, S.S., Phillips, R.S., Davis, R.B., *et al.* (2008) 'Patient expectations as predictors of outcome in patients with acute low back pain.' *J. Gen. Intern. Med. 23*, 148–153.

Paley, C.A., Johnson, M.I., Tashani, O.A., and Bagnall, A.M. (2012) 'Acupuncture for cancer pain in adults.' *Cochrane Database of Systematic Reviews 1*, CD007753.

Pennick, V., and Liddle, S.D. (2013) 'Interventions for preventing and treating pelvic and back pain in pregnancy.' *Cochrane Database of Systematic Reviews 8*, CD001139.

Ross, J., White, A., and Ernst, E. (1999) 'Western, minimal acupuncture for neck pain: a cohort study.' *Acupunct. Med. 17*, 1, 5–8.

Scharf, H.P., Mansmann, U., Streitberger, K., *et al.* (2006) 'Acupuncture and knee osteoarthritis: a three-armed randomized trial.' *Ann. Intern. Med. 145*, 12–20.

Sherman, K.J. (2014) 'The benefits of acupuncture: what you think is what you get, or is it?' *Acupunct. Med. 32*, 1, 2–3.

Sherman, K.J., Cherkin, D.C., Ichikawa, L., *et al.* (2010) 'Treatment expectations and preferences as predictors of outcome of acupuncture for chronic back pain.' *Spine 35*, 1471–1477.

Stomski, N.J., Mackintosh, S.F., and Stanley, M. (2014) 'The experience of acupuncture care from the perspective of people with chronic low back pain: a grounded theory study.' *Acupunct. Med. 32*, 333–339.

Thomas, K.J., MacPherson, H., Thorpe, L., *et al.* (2006) 'Randomized controlled trial of a short course of traditional acupuncture compared with usual care for persistent non-specific low back pain.' *BMJ 333*, 623.

Trigkilidas, D. (2010) 'Acupuncture therapy for chronic lower back pain: a systematic review.' *Ann. R. Coll. Surg. Engl. 92*, 595–598.

Trinh, K., Graham, N., Gross, A., *et al.* (2006) 'Acupuncture for neck disorders.' *Cochrane Database of Systematic Reviews 3*, CD004870.

Vas, J., Ortega, C., Olmo, V., *et al.* (2008) 'Single-point acupuncture and physiotherapy for the treatment of painful shoulder: a multicentre randomized controlled trial.' *Rheumatology 47*, 887–893.

Vickers, A.J., and Zollman, C. (1999) 'ABC of complementary medicine: acupuncture. Clinical review.' *BMJ 319*, 973–976.

Vickers, A.J., Cronin, A.M., Maschino, A.C., *et al.* (2012) 'Acupuncture for chronic pain: individual patient data meta-analysis.' *Arch. Intern. Med. 172*, 19, 1444–1453.

Waumsley, C. (2015) *Acupuncture vs. Dry Needling – Commentary.* The Dry Needling Institute. Available at www.thedryneedlinginstitute.net/wp-content/uploads/2012/04/ACUPUNCTURE-VS-DRY-NEEDLING.pdf, accessed on 21 July 2015.

Weidong, L., and Rosenthal, D.S. (2013) 'Acupuncture for cancer pain and related symptoms.' *Curr. Pain Headache Rep. 17*, 3, 321.

White, A. (2009) 'Recent progress in clinical research of acupuncture.' *The Bulletin of Meiji University of Integrative Medicine*, 23–28.

White, A., Foster, N., Cummings, M., *et al.* (2006) 'The effectiveness of acupuncture for osteoarthritis of the knee – a systematic review.' *Acupunct. Med. 24 Suppl.*, S40–S48.

White, A., Richardson, M., Richmond, P., Freedman, J., and Bevis, M. (2012) 'Group acupuncture for knee pain: evaluation of a cost-saving initiative in the health service.' *Acupunct. Med. 30*, 170–175.

WISCA (2015) *The Illegal and Unsafe Practice of Acupuncture Under the Term 'Dry Needling': 10 Facts You Should Know.* Wisconsin Society of Certified Acupuncturists. Available at http://acupuncturewisconsin.org/dry-needling-10-facts-you-should-know-2, accessed on 21 July 2015.

Witt, C.M., Brinkhaus, B., Jena, S., *et al.* (2005) 'Acupuncture in patients with osteoarthritis of the knee: a randomised trial.' *Lancet 366*, 136–143.

Witt, C.M., Jena, S., Brinkhaus, B., *et al.* (2006a) 'Acupuncture for patients with chronic neck pain.' *Pain 125*, 98–106.

Witt, C.M., Jena, S., Selim, D., *et al.* (2006b) 'Pragmatic randomized trial evaluating the clinical and economic effectiveness of acupuncture for chronic low back pain.' *American Journal of Epidemiology 164*, 487–496.

Part III

PREPARING FOR TREATMENT

Chapter 7

Safety Aspects of Dry Needling

Introduction to dry needling

Acupuncture is an ancient Chinese system of medicine in which fine needles are inserted at strategic sites in the body for preventive or therapeutic purposes (Stux, Berman and Pomeranz 2007). Because of its traditional origin, it is often seen as a form of complementary or alternative medicine (CAM). However, acupuncture is now widely used throughout Western countries, including the UK and USA (Zhang 2002); more and more patients are turning to acupuncture for treatment of many chronic conditions that conventional treatments have been unable to treat (VanderPloeg and Yi 2009).

Dry needling, also known as Western medical acupuncture (WMA), rationalizes an unbiased scientific evaluation of its role in a modern health service (Zhang 2002). This differentiates it from traditional Chinese medicine (TCM), since TCM is based on the belief that an energy, or 'life force' (qi), flows through a system of channels in the body, called meridians (Pyne and Shenker 2008). White and the Editorial Board of Acupuncture in Medicine (2009) suggest that WMA is based on a variety of neurophysiological concepts: stimulation of the central and peripheral nervous systems and the release of various pain-modulating substances, such as endorphins, substance P and calcitonin gene-related peptide (CGRP), to name a few. Conversely, traditional practitioners believe that the abnormalities in the flow of qi lead to illness, and that acupuncture restores health through restoration of this flow (VanderPloeg and Yi 2009).

Acupuncture is typically performed after an assessment of the patient's medical history, general health and a physical examination, followed by placing of the acupuncture needles at the acupuncture points that lasts between 20 and 40 minutes (Campbell 1999). This procedure may be repeated to achieve the desired end results. The procedure is conducted in a standing or sitting position, with some or all of the patient's clothing removed to access the required body part. Typically, fine single-use, pre-sterilized needles of a few inches in length are placed on the acupoints during a session. Once in place, these are left to act for a period of a few to 30 minutes. The subject may feel a tingling sensation or a dull ache during needle insertion (Lundeberg 2013).

The World Health Organization (1999) recommends that appropriate care should be taken during needling insertion. The needling should never reach the level of pain. If it becomes uncomfortable or painful for the patient, it should be stopped, depending on the severity. In addition, the needles should not be moved abruptly, since this may result in them becoming displaced or lost.

Medical uses of acupuncture

Acupuncture has a wide variety of clinical applications. According to a review by the World Health Organization (2002), numerous controlled trials have reported acupuncture as an effective intervention for various symptoms or conditions. However, the most widespread use of the therapy is for pain management, most commonly musculoskeletal pain (White and the Editorial Board of Acupuncture in Medicine 2009). Kaptchuk (2002) stated that a reasonable number of studies on acupuncture confirmed its analgesic effect in diverse pain conditions, although the author also mentioned that many studies did not find conclusive evidence for acupuncture in other conditions.

The conditions for which acupuncture is supported by controlled trials are:

- Myofascial pain

- Headache

- Menstrual cramps

- Induction of labour

- Knee pain

- Low back pain

- Sciatica

- Periarthritis of shoulder

- Carpal tunnel syndrome

- Post-operative pain

- Tennis elbow

- Leukopenia

- Rheumatoid arthritis

- Renal colic

(Lee, LaRiccia and Newberg 2004; Ulett, Han and
Han 1998; World Health Organization 2002)

The National Institute for Health and Care Excellence (NICE) provides guidelines for the use of acupuncture in the UK. Currently, only three conditions (persistent lower back pain, chronic tension-type headaches and migraines) have been recommended for treatment with acupuncture (NHS Choices 2015).

Apart from these, many practitioners have found acupuncture useful in a wide range of medical conditions, including post-operative nausea and vomiting, allergies, hay fever, eczema, fatigue, depression and anxiety, digestive disorders, irritable bowel syndrome (IBS), infertility and menstrual disorders, insomnia and dry mouth (xerostomia) (Beyens 1993). However, thorough medical evidence is either lacking or inconclusive to support the use of acupuncture in many of these conditions (see Table 7.1).

Adverse effects of dry needling

A number of published studies have provided reassuring confirmation about the safety of medical acupuncture. According to Lee *et al.* (2004), studies done to evaluate the safety of acupuncture found only nine reported incidents about licensed acupuncturists and 50 adverse events over a 20-year period. In addition, several published systematic reviews of adverse events linked with acupuncture concluded that, on rare occasions, acupuncture could induce the complications related to any type of needle use (Bensoussan, Myers and Carlton 2000; Peuker *et al.* 1999; Yamashita *et al.* 2001).

Table 7.1 Findings of systematic reviews and meta-analyses of acupuncture for conditions related to pain

Condition	Study (reference)	RCTs*, n	Findings	Conclusions
Post-operative pain	Sun et al. (2008)	15	Nine studies reported a statistically significant reduction in pain scores compared with control groups, one study was excluded from the analysis and three studies did not report data on pain scores.	Peri-operative acupuncture may be a useful adjunct for post-operative analgesia.
Acute dental pain	Ernst and Pittler (1998)	16	Twelve trials reported that acupuncture was more effective than controls, but four trials suggested the contrary.	Acupuncture can reduce dental pain.
Low back pain	Furlan et al. (2005)	35	The average improvement in pain with acupuncture for acute low back pain was 52% (based on two studies), 32% for chronic (16 studies) and 51% for unknown or mixed durations of pain (eight studies).	Acupuncture is more effective than sham or no treatment; appears to be useful adjunct to other therapies for chronic low back pain.
Myofascial trigger point (MTrP) pain	Tough and White (2011)	7	Six studies reported statistically superior outcomes compared to placebo.	Acupuncture is superior to placebo; is likely to be the most effective approach for MTrP-derived pain.
Fibromyalgia	Berman et al. (1999)	3	All the trials found statistically significant positive findings compared with control groups.	Acupuncture may be effective for fibromyalgia; more high-quality trials are needed.
Osteoarthritis of the knee	Ezzo et al. (2001)	7†	Two trials compared acupuncture with wait list: both found statistically significant results; three trials compared acupuncture to placebo: two found statistically significant outcomes; two trials compared acupuncture to physical therapy: both reported no significant finding for acupuncture.	Acupuncture may play a role in the treatment of knee osteoarthritis; more well-designed trials are necessary to reach a conclusive decision.

* *RCT = randomized, controlled trial.*

† *Review and analysis contain some trials that were not randomized.*

In prospective studies, acupuncture is also established as a very safe intervention for patients. A prospective study of adverse effects following 34,000 consultations with professional acupuncturists registered with the British Acupuncture Council revealed that only about 1.1 cases per 10,000 consultations led to serious effects such as hospital admission, prolonged hospital stays, permanent disability or death (MacPherson *et al.* 2001). Minor adverse events were recorded in 0.13 per cent of patients, and mild transient reactions were recorded in 15 per cent of patients. However, the most common mild transient reactions were feeling normal and feeling energized, which are in fact positive and desired effects (MacPherson *et al.* 2001). Another prospective national survey done by MacPherson *et al.* (2004) also suggested that the incidence of side effects related to acupuncture is relatively rare.

Although some studies have reported blood-borne diseases such as hepatitis and HIV, they are negligible, since disposable needles are now widely used. Other side effects reported include bleeding, infection, broken needles, punctures of organs, cardiac tamponade, nerve damage and contact dermatitis (Kaptchuk 2002). However, it is now well-established that many of these adverse events usually occur when acupuncturists have inadequate training (White *et al.* 2001).

Conversely, Cummings (2011) suggests that there are some mild, temporary adverse reactions of acupuncture which may occur in some cases despite the proper administration of acupuncture by a qualified practitioner. These include:

- pain at the point of needle puncture

- bleeding or bruising from the puncture point

- drowsiness

- feeling unwell

- dizziness or fainting

- worsening of pre-existing symptoms.

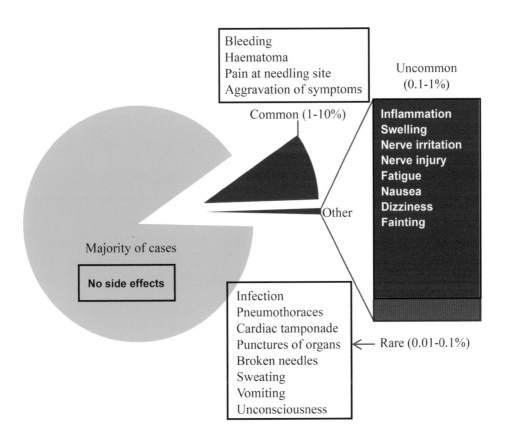

Figure 7.1 Reported side effects of acupuncture (derived from the statistical findings of Vincent 2001; White 2006; Witt et al. 2009; Zhao et al. 2011)

Guidelines for the monitoring of accidents and untoward reactions

The World Health Organization (1999) has recommended the following adverse effects to be monitored during acupuncture treatments.

Fainting

Fainting is uncommon; however, it could occur during the first session (MacPherson *et al.* 2001). Hence, the patient needs to be informed properly, and the procedure needs to be conducted in a position where the patient can be comfortable. Symptoms of impending faintness include feeling unwell, difficulty breathing, dizziness, the room moving, a feeling of weakness and a restricted feeling in the chest accompanied by palpitations, nausea or vomiting. Furthermore, the complexion may turn pale, and the pulse may become weak and irregular. All the needles must be removed immediately on appearance of these warning symptoms. The symptoms often disappear after a short rest. In addition, the fainting episodes occur most commonly in a fasted subject and can be avoided by ensuring that the patient has taken a proper meal before acupuncture (Zhao *et al.* 2011).

In the event that the patient faints, first aid procedures as provided by HSE (2011) should be followed to help the patient recover from the incident. In most cases, the patient revives without any emergency medical treatment. However, if the patient does not regain consciousness within two minutes, the practitioner should carry out conventional testing and may call for emergency medical help, depending on the severity of the patient's condition. At the same time, the practitioner should carefully roll the patient on their side so that they are supported by one leg and one arm, bend the top leg so both hip and knee are at right angles, open their airway by leaning their head back and raising their chin, and monitor their breathing and pulse continuously (Abe *et al.* 2009).

Needle shock

This occurs in about 1.3 per cent of the subjects (MacPherson *et al.* 2001) and is a vaso-vagal response characterized by light-headedness, general malaise, cold perspiration, nausea, chest tightness and, in extreme situations, unconsciousness (Hamilton 1995). On appearance of any of these symptoms, all the needles must be removed immediately and the patient monitored closely. Though rare, this should be noted as an adverse event in the records and proper treatment should be followed. Needle shock may be avoided in a number of ways. These include treating patients in the lying position, needling gently as a test dose, reassuring nervous patients, ensuring the patient is not over-tired or hungry, and avoiding needling the thoracic area over the sympathetic chain (especially if the patient is anxious or fearful).

Bleeding

Any bleeding or effusion of body fluids should be treated in accordance with medical guidelines. The spills should be cleaned with a disinfectant agent (RCN 2013).

Drowsiness

Some patients may feel very relaxed and even sleepy after acupuncture treatment. They should be advised not to drive until they have fully recovered (World Health Organization 1999).

Broken needle

The incidence of broken needles with acupuncture is very rare (White 2004). In a prospective survey of 139,988 acupuncture treatments, Umlauf (1988) reported only two incidents of broken needles. However, in rare cases, a tip may break off and remain in the patient. If the needle breaks, the patient should be reassured and the broken tip should be removed with forceps. If it is not possible to retrieve the tip, the area should be marked and detailed notes should be prepared, followed by referring the patient to the concerned department (World Health Organization 1999).

Stuck needle

If a needle is stuck, the practitioner should reassure the patient and encourage him/her to become relaxed. All the other needles should be carefully removed, and gentle massage should be employed to retrieve the stuck needle.

Needle stick injury

Also referred to as percutaneous injury, this needs care to avoid infections. Although rare, injuries from sharps contaminated with an infected patient's blood can transmit any of more than 20 diseases, including Hepatitis B and C and human immunodeficiency virus (HIV). Immediate action is advised to encourage the wound to gently bleed, ideally by holding it under running water, followed by first aid and medical care and post-exposure prophylaxis (HSE 2013; RCN 2013).

Risk of transmission of a blood-borne virus (BBV)

Although the use of gloves has been shown to reduce the risk of transmission of infection, owing to reduced manual dexterity they are not used except when it is known that the patient is carrying a blood-borne infection.

Percutaneous injuries carry the greatest risk of exposure to and transmission of BBVs in the healthcare setting. The highest risks of injuries are in hospital wards, operating theatres and A&E units (Health Protection Agency *et al.* 2012). The risk of infection from a BBV following a percutaneous injury within the healthcare setting has been estimated as 1 in 3 for Hepatitis B, 1 in 30 for Hepatitis C and 1 in 300 for HIV (Health Protection Agency *et al.* 2012).

Safety and regulation of dry needling

In many countries, including the United Kingdom, there is no statutory regulation of acupuncture, but many non-medical acupuncturists are required to register with their local authority. This is because of the risk of blood-borne infections from piercing the skin with acupuncture needles (White 2004). The same rules also cover tattooing and body piercing. Hence, the local authority is responsible for formulating the bylaws that govern the cleanliness of the acupuncture premises, practitioners, instruments, materials and equipment.

In addition, a number of nations have independent organizations which an acupuncture practitioner can join. These organizations usually require a minimum qualification and certain codes of practice to be followed. In the United Kingdom, acupuncture organizations include the:

- British Medical Acupuncture Society (BMAS)

- Acupuncture Association of Chartered Physiotherapists (AACP)

- British Acupuncture Council (BacC)

- British Academy of Western Medical Acupuncture (BAWMA)

- British Register of Complementary Practitioners (BRCP).

In general, the codes of practice of these organizations prescribe the following achievable targets:

- *The workplace* must be suitable for carrying out professional medical work of this kind. The premises must be capable of being kept clean; used solely for acupuncture practice or other similar work; have sufficient sanitary facilities for all users of the clinic/practice; and meet current fire precaution and health and safety standards. If a private home is used, the treatment room(s) must not be used for any ordinary domestic purposes.

Suitable hand-washing facilities should be available. This facility should have a washbasin with a clean-running hot water supply, preferably wrist, arm or foot operated. This should be for the sole use of the practitioners and other involved staff. This must be located in or in the near vicinity of (i.e. not necessitating the opening and closing of doors with your hands) the treatment room. It must also have: liquid soap dispenser; disposable paper towels; and an adequately sized bin, pedal operated if lidded, situated near the basin.

The treatment room must allow free movement and easy cleaning. It must have: sufficient space to allow free movement and establish a clean field; sufficient storage; smooth, easily cleanable surfaces on tabletops, shelves and all working surfaces; smooth, impervious surfaces on treatment couches or other furniture used for treatment; smooth, impervious flooring or short pile (not looped) commercial carpeting; and adequate heating, ventilation and artificial lighting.

The practitioner must avoid possible cross-infection of treatment surfaces. Surfaces should be covered with fresh paper couch roll, disposed of after treating each patient. If covering is with towels or sheets alone, these must be fresh for each patient and boiled or machine-washed on the 40–60 degrees setting before being reused. All surfaces must be regularly cleaned with an appropriate detergent, at the very least at the beginning or end of every working day. If any spillage of blood or body fluids occurs during treatment, soiled items must be placed in yellow clinical waste bags at the end of the treatment session.

The treatment room must be kept clean. At least weekly, all tabletops, shelves and impervious surfaces must be cleaned and dusted; all impervious floor surfaces must be washed daily with appropriate cleansers; all carpets in the areas adjacent to treatment surfaces must be vacuum-cleaned daily and annually steam-cleaned; and all blankets used in treatment must be frequently laundered.

- *Equipment.* Equipment that conforms to the current guidelines should be used. One must use:

  » single-use, pre-sterilized, disposable solid needles, which, if in multipacks of five, ten or more needles, must not be used or stored for use after the session in which the seal on the package is broken; any needle with a damaged packaging seal must not be used

» pre-packaged sterile guide tubes with each individual needle or set of needles; they must not be used or stored for use beyond the treatment session in which the seal on the package is broken

» pre-sterilized, single-use plum blossom needles ('seven star hammers')

» single-use paper tissues, paper towels and couch roll

» disinfectants: for skin disinfection pre-packaged 70 per cent isopropyl alcohol swabs with or without 0.5%–2.0% chlorhexidine must be used; for impervious room surfaces any reliable branded product is adequate

» sterile cotton wool and non-sterile cotton wool/buds

» disposable surgical gloves

» sharps box conforming to BS 7320:1990 and clearly marked 'Danger – Contaminated Needles – To Be Incinerated' (Department of Health 2013)

» a first aid kit complying with BS 8599 (HSE 2014).

• *Duty of care.* The practitioner must ensure the health and safety of the patient. The patient's known medical history and potential allergic reactions must be taken account of. The part of the body to be treated should be clean, and must be free of any cuts or wounds. Any paper or other material used as a covering, and any towel, cloth or other article which is applied to the patient's skin, should be clean and should not have been used in connection with any other patient unless thoroughly disinfected before use.

Unattended patients should be asked to avoid movements that could cause them injury through bending or damaging a needle; ensure that they can call you immediately at any time.

In case a patient has, or is suspected of having, an infectious disease or serious pre-existing medical condition, the practitioner must ensure that it is safe to treat them by contacting their GP if necessary. Although treatment may be offered, the patient should be advised not to view acupuncture as a substitute for any treatment for a notifiable disease that a doctor has prescribed.

The practitioner must ensure that their own health and personal hygiene do not endanger the health of patients. Any cuts and wounds must be covered with a waterproof dressing; nails must be kept short and clean; suitable clean clothing must be worn, without large, loose or dangling jewellery or rings; and giving treatment must be avoided when suffering from an infectious or contagious condition that may be transmitted to the patient. The practitioner should inform their general practitioner as soon as possible if a suspicion of suffering from or having been in contact with someone suffering from a notifiable infectious disease arises.

- *Responsibility of the practitioner.* The practitioner must wash their hands thoroughly with liquid soap and warm water immediately before any acupuncture procedure and ensure that a clean field is established. Hands must be dried with a clean disposable towel. Alcohol hand-rub gel or foam is not a substitute for hand-washing at this stage of the treatment.

The practitioner must insert needles hygienically and safely, by ensuring the following safety aspects:

» The skin at the needle site is clean.

» Any areas of the body where moisture or exudates may collect are swabbed clean with an alcohol swab before needling.

» All single-use, pre-sterilized needles and instruments are opened in the patient's presence immediately before use.

» A fresh needle is used for every point needled during a session.

» The shaft of the needle is never touched with bare fingers or with non-sterile materials. The practitioner must not place a needle on an intermediate surface before use and must use only sterile material to support the shaft of the needle once it has been inserted or if it is inserted without a guide tube.

The hands are to be properly cleansed again if at any time during treatment they are contaminated by contact with clothing, pens, clinic furniture, etc. between separate needle insertions.

The practitioner must wear well-fitting disposable surgical gloves if:

» blood or body fluid is spilled, which must be cleaned up promptly with detergent and followed up with disinfectant solution

» the patient has open lesions or is known to have a contagious disease

» the practitioner has cuts or wounds on their hands which cannot be covered adequately by a waterproof dressing or has a skin infection

» the practitioner is handling blood-soiled items, body fluids, excretions and secretions, as well as the surfaces, materials and objects exposed to them.

The practitioner must remove needles hygienically and safely and place each needle immediately into the sharps container. While drawing blood, light pressure should be applied with clean cotton wool or a clean swab, avoiding contact with the patient's body fluids, and the cotton wool or swab disposed of immediately in a sharps container or clinical waste bag.

On needling a point, the practitioner must not re-palpate the point with their bare finger during that treatment session unless the fingertips have been cleansed by hand-washing or by the use of alcohol gel. The hands must be washed thoroughly at the end of treatment to reduce the risk of cross-infection with the subsequent patient.

- *Personal safety.* The practitioner should act promptly on suffering a needle stick injury by encouraging free bleeding from the site; washing thoroughly with soap and water but without scrubbing; and seeking medical advice immediately, preferably within one hour (Government of UK 1999).

- *Disposal of equipment and clinical waste.* The practitioner should dispose of used equipment and clinical waste safely, by placing all needles immediately after use in appropriate sharps disposal containers and disposing of the containers in accordance with Department of Health (2013) guidelines.

The practitioner must dispose of all clinical waste that has been contaminated with the spillage of body fluids such as blood, open wound abrasions or mucous membranes in sealed clinical waste bags collected by a licensed agent. All contracts and receipts for clinical waste collection should be maintained.

The practitioner should dispose of all other waste that has not come into contact with body fluids or spillages, including needle wrappings and single-use guide tubes, as commercial or domestic waste, provided that it is carefully double-bagged daily (Department of Health 2013).

- *Home visits.* The practitioner using a mobile practice or undertaking home visits must meet health and safety standards equivalent to working in a clinic. There must be a defined base of at least one room within home or business premises containing adequate facilities for the disinfection of equipment (if appropriate), the storage of clean equipment and the temporary storage of soiled equipment, clinical waste and sharps containers.

  During the transport of equipment, containers used for this purpose must be of sufficient size, designed to allow for the separate storage of sterile and soiled equipment, and lockable and tightly sealed when shut.

  During treatments at a patient's home, it should be ensured that the treatment is carried out in a well-lit, clean room with ready access to a clean wash-hand basin. The practitioner should carry appropriate cleaning agents, hand disinfectants and a hygienic means of hand drying; carry clean couch rolls and paper towels for covering work surfaces in the home and ensure that the bed/couch is covered by a clean cover; and in all cases ensure a clean field is established. After treatment is completed, the practitioner must ensure that used needles are discarded immediately in a portable sharps container; any soiled or contaminated non-sharps items are disposed of in the appropriate manner; and other waste products are carefully bagged separately for disposal in line with local environmental health department guidelines.

  The practitioner must also set aside sufficient time before leaving to ensure that the patient is experiencing no adverse reactions to treatment and is well enough for the practitioner to leave.

- *Maintaining records.* The practitioner must maintain a permanent attendance register which records all patients attending the clinic and which links to a written record of their contact details.

- *Commitment to health and safety.* The practitioner must comply with the requirements and provisions of Health and Safety at Work legislation (Government of UK 1999). The duty of care extends not only to patients and employees but also to the general public and visitors to the premises. All major accidents to employees and members of the public must be reported in accordance with the provisions of the Reporting of Injuries, Diseases and Dangerous Occurrences Regulations (RIDDOR) (Government of UK 2013). Furthermore, the practitioner must check that: all floors, passages and stairs are kept free from obstruction; equipment and machinery is regularly inspected and maintained; and all electrical and gas appliances are regularly examined.

Special precautions with difficult and dangerous acupoints

Some of the acupoints are difficult to access owing to their location (Grant and Ma 2003). A professional with a suboptimal understanding of such acupoints may endanger the patient. The most important factors that can minimize the danger are proper monitoring of the angle of insertion and depth of penetration.

In addition to general precautions observed during medical procedures, acupuncture warrants additional precaution measures for the safety of the patient (Chou, Chu and Lin 2011). The practitioner needs to have a thorough understanding of the anatomical features of the insertion site and its variation with age and pathological conditions. As a rule of thumb, insertion sites that are in close proximity to vital organs and sensitive structures, including the vertex of skull, occipital area, frontal and temporal area, intercostal spaces and suprasternal area, vertebral column and sacrum, need to be handled with absolute precision (World Health Organization 1999). The depth of the insertion site needs to be based on clinical examination of the patient's morphology and local anatomy (Chou *et al.* 2011).

Conclusion

From consideration of the above guidelines and from analysing reports of accidents with acupuncture, it can be concluded that the risk of adverse events associated with acupuncture is very low, lower than many of the conventional medical treatments. Besides, most of the acupuncture side effects are transient and disappear without the need for intervention. However, even if acupuncture is so demonstrably safe, a practitioner needs to be cautious for the patient's benefit and should be concerned that unexpected accidents may occur.

Serious events related to acupuncture are avoidable, since many are caused by the malpractice of acupuncturists. However, Grant and Ma (2003) suggested some potential risk factors of acupuncture that are linked with the occurrence of incidents. These include:

- insufficient education or training in acupuncture

- incomplete knowledge of human anatomy and histology or of certain physiological or pathological conditions

- failure to check for abnormal anatomy

- poor needling technique (depth and angle or stimulating too strongly)

- not paying attention to the patient's past medical history and existing condition.

The authors also noted that, by avoidance of these risk factors, the safety of acupuncture could be ensured.

References

Abe, H., Benditt, D.G., Decker, W.W., Grubb, B.P., Sheldon, R., and Shen, W.K. (2009) 'Guidelines for the diagnosis and management of syncope (version 2009).' *European Heart Journal 30*, 2631–2671.

Bensoussan, A., Myers, S.P., and Carlton, A.L. (2000) 'Risks associated with the practice of traditional Chinese medicine: an Australian study.' *Archives of Family Medicine 9*, 10, 1071.

Berman, B.M., Ezzo, J., Hadhazy, V., and Swyers, J.P. (1999) 'Is acupuncture effective in the treatment of fibromyalgia?' *Journal of Family Practice 48*, 3, 213–218.

Beyens, F. (1993) 'Chinese acupuncture and moxibustion.' *Acupunct. Med. 11*, 2, 105–106.

Campbell, A. (1999) 'Acupuncture: where to place the needles and for how long.' *Acupunct. Med. 17*, 2, 113–117.

Chou, P.C., Chu, H.Y., and Lin, J.G. (2011) 'Safe needling depth of acupuncture points.' *Journal of Alternative and Complementary Medicine 17*, 3, 199–206.

Cummings, M. (2011) 'Safety aspects of electroacupuncture.' *Acupunct. Med. 29*, 2, 83–85.

Department of Health (2013) *Health Technical Memorandum 07-01: Safe Management of Healthcare Waste.* Available at www.gov.uk/government/uploads/system/uploads/attachment_data/file/167976/HTM_07-01_Final.pdf, accessed on 22 July 2015.

Ernst, E., and Pittler, M.H. (1998) 'The effectiveness of acupuncture in treating acute dental pain: a systematic review.' *British Dental Journal 184*, 9, 443–447.

Ezzo, J., Hadhazy, V., Birch, S., *et al.* (2001) 'Acupuncture for osteoarthritis of the knee: a systematic review.' *Arthritis & Rheumatism 44*, 4, 819–825.

Furlan, A.D., van Tulder, M.W., Cherkin, D.C., Tsukayama, H., Lao, L., Koes, B.W., and Berman, B.M. (2005) 'Acupuncture and dry-needling for low back pain.' *Cochrane Database of Systematic Reviews 1*, CD001351.

Government of UK (1999) *The Management of Health and Safety at Work Regulations 1999.* London: HMSO. Available at www.legislation.gov.uk/uksi/1999/3242/contents/made, accessed on 22 July 2015.

Government of UK (2013) *The Reporting of Injuries, Diseases and Dangerous Occurrences Regulations 2013.* London: HMSO. Available at www.legislation.gov.uk/uksi/2013/1471/contents/made, accessed on 22 July 2015.

Grant, A., and Ma, B.Y. (2003) 'The safe use of difficult and dangerous acupuncture points.' *Journal of Chinese Medicine 72*, 11–15.

Hamilton, J.G. (1995) 'Needle phobia: a neglected diagnosis.' *Journal of Family Practice 41*, 2, 169–175.

Health Protection Agency, Health Protection Services; Public Health Wales; Public Health Agency Northern Ireland; Health Protection Scotland (2012) *Eye of the Needle: United Kingdom Surveillance of Significant Occupational Exposure to Bloodborne Viruses in Healthcare Workers.* London: Health Protection Agency.

HSE (2011) *Basic Advice on First Aid at Work.* London: Health and Safety Executive. Available at www.hse.gov.uk/pubns/indg347.pdf, accessed on 22 July 2015.

HSE (2013) *Health and Safety (Sharp Instruments in Healthcare) Regulations.* London: Health and Safety Executive. Available at www.hse.gov.uk/pubns/hsis7.pdf, accessed on 22 July 2015.

HSE (2014) *First Aid at Work: Your Questions Answered.* London: Health and Safety Executive. Available at www.hse.gov.uk/pubns/indg214.pdf, accessed on 22 July 2015.

Kaptchuk, T.J. (2002) 'Acupuncture: theory, efficacy, and practice.' *Annals of Internal Medicine 136*, 5, 374–383.

Lee, B.Y., LaRiccia, P.J., and Newberg, A.B. (2004) 'Acupuncture in theory and practice. Part 2: Clinical indications, efficacy, and safety.' *Hospital Physician 40*, 5, 33–38.

Lundeberg, T. (2013) 'Mechanisms of Acupuncture in Pain: A Physiological Perspective in a Clinical Context.' In H. Hong (ed.) *Acupuncture: Theories and Evidence.* Singapore: World Scientific. Available at http://media.axon.es/pdf/97162_1.pdf, accessed on 22 July 2015.

MacPherson, H., Scullion, A., Thomas, K.J., and Walters, S. (2004) 'Patient reports of adverse events associated with acupuncture treatment: a prospective national survey.' *Quality and Safety in Health Care 13*, 5, 349–355.

MacPherson, H., Thomas, K., Walters, S., and Fitter, M. (2001) 'A prospective survey of adverse events and treatment reactions following 34,000 consultations with professional acupuncturists.' *Acupunct. Med. 19*, 2, 93–102.

NHS Choices (2015) *Acupuncture.* Available at www.nhs.uk/conditions/acupuncture/Pages/Introduction.aspx, accessed on 21 July 2015.

Peuker, E.T., White, A., Ernst, E., Pera, F., and Filler, T.J. (1999) 'Traumatic complications of acupuncture: therapists need to know human anatomy.' *Archives of Family Medicine 8*, 6, 553.

Pyne, D., and Shenker, N.G. (2008) 'Demystifying acupuncture.' *Rheumatology 47*, 8, 1132–1136.

RCN (2013) *Sharps Safety: RCN Guidance to Support the Implementation of The Health and Safety (Sharp Instruments in Healthcare) Regulations 2013.* London: Royal College of Nursing. Available at www.rcn.org.uk/__data/assets/pdf_file/0008/418490/004135.pdf, accessed on 22 July 2015.

Stux, G., Berman, B., and Pomeranz, B. (2007) *Basics of Acupuncture* (fifth edition). Berlin and Heidelberg: Springer.

Sun, Y., Gan, T.J., Dubose, J.W., and Habib, A.S. (2008) 'Acupuncture and related techniques for postoperative pain: a systematic review of randomized controlled trials.' *British Journal of Anaesthesia 101*, 2, 151–160.

Tough, E.A., and White, A.R. (2011) 'Effectiveness of acupuncture/dry needling for myofascial trigger point pain.' *Physical Therapy Reviews 16*, 2, 147–154.

Ulett, G.A., Han, J., and Han, S. (1998) 'Traditional and evidence-based acupuncture.' *Southern Medical Journal 91*, 12, 1115–1120.

Umlauf, R. (1988) 'Analysis of the main results of the activity of the acupuncture department of faculty hospital.' *Acupuncture in Medicine 5*, 2, 16–18.

VanderPloeg, K., and Yi, X. (2009) 'Acupuncture in modern society.' *Journal of Acupuncture and Meridian Studies 2*, 1, 26–33.

Vincent, C. (2001) 'The safety of acupuncture: acupuncture is safe in the hands of competent practitioners.' *British Medical Journal 323*, 7311, 467.

White, A. (2004) 'A cumulative review of the range and incidence of significant adverse events associated with acupuncture.' *Acupunct. Med. 22*, 3, 122–133.

White, A. (2006) 'The safety of acupuncture – evidence from the UK.' *Acupunct. Med. 24 (Suppl.)*, 53–57.

White, A., and the Editorial Board of Acupuncture in Medicine (2009) 'Western medical acupuncture: a definition.' *Acupunct. Med. 27*, 1, 33.

White, A., Hayhoe, S., Hart, A., and Ernst, E. (2001) 'Survey of adverse events following acupuncture (SAFA): a prospective study of 32,000 consultations.' *Acupunct. Med. 19*, 2, 84–92.

Witt, C.M., Pach, D., Brinkhaus, B., *et al.* (2009) 'Safety of acupuncture: results of a prospective observational study with 229,230 patients and introduction of a medical information and consent form.' *Forschende Komplementärmedizin/Research in Complementary Medicine 16*, 2, 91–97.

World Health Organization (1999) *Guidelines on Basic Training and Safety in Acupuncture.* Available at http://whqlibdoc.who.int/hq/1999/WHO_EDM_TRM_99.1.pdf, accessed on 22 July 2015.

World Health Organization (2002) *Acupuncture: Review and Analysis of Reports on Controlled Clinical Trials.* Available at http://whqlibdoc.who.int/publications/2002/9241545437.pdf, accessed on 22 July 2015.

Yamashita, H., Tsukayama, H., White, A.R., Tanno, Y., Sugishita, C., and Ernst, E. (2001) 'Systematic review of adverse events following acupuncture: the Japanese literature.' *Complementary Therapies in Medicine 9*, 2, 98–104.

Zhang, G. (2002) 'Acupuncture and moxibustion.' *Contemporary Chinese Medicine and Acupuncture 2002*, 60–83.

Zhao, L., Zhang, F.W., Li, Y., *et al.* (2011) 'Adverse events associated with acupuncture: three multicentre randomized controlled trials of 1968 cases in China.' *Trials 12*, 1, 87.

Chapter 8

Palpation

It is assumed that the reader has some experience of palpation. However, it is a subject always worth revisiting as there is no limit to how much you can improve your technique (Denmei 2003). Palpation is the practice of informed touch. It is both an art and science and requires skills, dedication and practice. It needs to be performed with sensitivity, as we are palpating human beings who are often in pain and discomfort and who are seeking professional help. There is no substitute for good palpation, and with practice one can have confidence in knowing what is normal and abnormal. With time one can develop reliable, rapid, responsive instruments.

The muscular system can be evaluated in a number of ways, including strength, movement, appearance, tone, firing patterns, and active and passive movements. Palpation is just one of those means of investigation, but is an important one. Czechoslovakian Dr Vladimir Janda emphasized the fact that time spent in assessment will save time in treatment (Janda 2012).

There has always been doubt raised over the reliability of palpation of musculoskeletal disorders; however, in daily practice it is used frequently. Finando and Finando (2005) describe palpation as a skill that is at the very core of manual therapy and helps us evaluate our patients and perhaps how patients evaluate the practitioner, as it is through the first touch that the patient discovers much about the practitioner and is part of the dialogue between patient and practitioner.

Radiography, MRI and other diagnostic tests and their interpretation are also part science and part art, so are no different from palpation, interpretation and reliability in some respects. However, whilst it is routine and best practice to send patients for further diagnostic scans, there is debate as to how informative the results are, as up to 60 per cent of women and 80 per cent of men at age 50 show evidence of degenerative changes of the spinal column, while by the age of 70 the figure is 95 per cent for both sexes.

When palpating, a detailed knowledge of anatomy, attachments, insertions and muscle action are all essential components. Generally speaking, healthy muscle tissue will feel soft, pliable and alive. Every muscle will have its own particular characteristics in terms of fibre orientation, action and typical areas where it will develop dysfunction. Every 'body' tells a story…let the body speak to you.

What we decide about the information from our palpation essentially has to be assimilated within each practitioner's professional context, whether osteopathy, chiropractic, physiotherapy, acupuncture or other profession, and used accordingly. Each practitioner has to use their own subjective description of what they are feeling and put that into a diagnostic framework. Dr Felix Mann, a well-known pioneer of Western acupuncture in the UK, commented that there is little if any part of the body surface that has not been designated to some therapeutic system (Mann 2000). This can be clearly seen within traditional Chinese medicine (TCM) with the 12 main channels, eight extra channels, extra points, scalp points and auricular points.

Palpation skills are fundamental as a diagnostic aid because they affect clinical results. A palpatory examination is essential when continuing to treat a patient because it confirms if any change has taken place which will change or reinforce our treatment strategies and protocols. However, palpation is a complex task that requires the right combination of knowledge, skills and attitude and can only be learnt by palpating on a regular basis.

A degree of sensitivity must be applied when palpating, as some patients have little or no body awareness and may have different cultural connotations. While the palpatory process will be second nature to the experienced practitioner, it may be a strange or unfamiliar process for the patient. This is in direct contrast to the more body-aware athletes or those who partake in regular physical activity who can often participate in the process and guide the practitioner.

MacPherson (1994, p.7) describes palpation as having an educational role 'whereby the patient learns to give weight and value to the subjective sensations of their body'. Sometimes palpation can validate what the patient is experiencing; or reveal to them that a distal unknown part of their body is capable of producing pain, as in cases of referred pain. Sometimes a technique can be performed for a few seconds and the same area re-palpated to detect for change to confirm to both patient and practitioner that a change has been made.

Technique

In discussing palpation, Legge (2011, p.36) states that 'each practitioner should develop their own way of developing a routine of examining each patient. Having a consistent structured approach for examination of each section is crucial to clinical success.' Aubin, Gagnon and Morin (2014) created the PALPATE acronym as a means of teaching osteopathy students the art of palpation. The results of this meant the students 'seemed more confident and, as predicted, demanded less external validation in technique classes. They understood more clearly the stakes of palpation and the importance of repeating each technical movement' (Aubin *et al.* 2014, p.8).

The seven steps are as follows:

1. Position – comfortable positioning of the clinician

2. Anatomy – 3D anatomic visualization

3. Level – depth of tissue contact

4. Purpose – clear identification of intention

5. Ascertain – initiate motion with a relative point of reference

6. Tweaking – fine-tuning of the five previous steps and perceptual exploration

7. Evaluate or normalize – apply technique parameters.

Another useful acronym commonly used is STAR or TART, developed by Dowling (1998), an osteopath who used the acronym for the findings of dysfunction in assessment and palpation:

Sensitivity

Tissue texture changes

Asymmetry

Range of motion reduced

or:

Tenderness

Asymmetry

Restricted motion

Tissue texture changes.

The process of palpation can be further categorized into static and motion palpation. In static palpation the patient is prone or supine and the practitioner will palpate the area or areas and observe what he/she feels. This is commonly used to detect areas of pain and tenderness. Motion palpation can be divided into active (non-practitioner-assisted) and passive (practitioner-assisted) and is used to assess functional movement that is normal for the patient being examined.

Palpation when searching for acupuncture points sometimes requires a very light touch and a focusing of your palpation skills. It is useful to alternate between the methods described for palpating trigger points, from a strong firm pressure to a lighter touch, as a lighter touch can be just as effective as a palpation tool. Denmei (2003) describes a number of methods for locating acupuncture points. These are areas and points with abnormal temperature, depressed points, points with abnormal moisture, and points with a feeling of softness like pressing on a balloon. Denmei further discusses other palpation techniques for locating points on the abdomen: using a stroking technique and pinching to detect changes in tissue and any abnormalities. Different areas vary, so a variety of palpation techniques should be employed to improve reliability.

Applicators

When considering the choice of applicators available, Neil-Asher (2014) describes using a number of different areas when palpating for trigger points. These are finger pads, flat finger, pincer palpation, flat hand, thenar eminence and elbow.

It must be stressed that not all areas of the body have equal amounts of touch receptors. The fingertips and tongue may have as many as 100 per cm^2; the back of the hand fewer than 10 per cm^2. Therefore, when palpating, the fingertips and thumb are the most sensitive areas, but with time one can develop sensitivity using different applicators.

Depth of pressure

Any pressure hard enough will result in pain, and is not very reliable as a clinical tool. Therefore vary the pressure, starting from light and increasing to moderate to deep. Light touch will include detections of change of skin temperature, moisture and elasticity. If you consider that soft tissue dysfunction can occur at any depth, then using a variable depth to probe the different layers is important.

Practitioner positioning is a key factor when palpating. Correct practitioner positioning can deliver varying forces and directions to the patient whilst maintaining practitioner comfort and awareness. Having the table set to a good working height should allow for the transference of bodyweight to the patient whilst being relaxed and not having hunched shoulders. Having the table/plinth too high usually results in increased muscular force being used to palpate deeper structures. This will result in loss of proprioception, increased strain and fatigue in the practitioner, and unnecessary force and pressure on the patient.

Structure and function

Structure and function are reciprocally interrelated. Functional demands involve demands from the structure to meet those needs.

To treat or not to treat – that is the question!

A tight hamstring may be stabilizing a dysfunctional sacroiliac joint, or it may be part of a larger clinical picture, such as Dr Vladimir Janda's lower-crossed syndrome (which is a particular pattern of muscular imbalance in the lower body).

Trigger points may be acting as stabilizing functions in hypermobile patients. Chaitow *et al.* (2010) hypothesize that trigger points have a functional purpose – to offer an efficient means of short-term stability in an otherwise unstable environment.

Faulty posture and its overload of the muscular system is now an extremely important factor in the patient population seen by manual therapists. Correcting faulty posture will often be a key part of the treatment strategy to relieve pain, highlighting the link between structure and function.

In reference to trigger points and the possible adaptations that can occur, Travell and Simons (1999) noted that trigger points in one area can affect the motor activity of other muscles. In one example it was seen that a trigger point in a right soleus caused a spasm in the right lumbar paraspinal muscles. Similarly, trigger points in the quadratus lumborum can cause inhibition of the ipsilateral gluteal muscles. No injury should be seen in isolation, and a full biomechanical assessment should always be performed.

Travell and Simons (1999), in their seminal work on trigger points, emphasized the importance of treating articular dysfunctions. A facilitated spinal segment can cause an increase in paraspinal activity. A trigger point and its associated increased tension can cause articular dysfunction, whilst simultaneously a facilitated spinal segment can contribute to trigger point activation via changes in the motor, sensory and autonomic components of the nervous system. This effect can occur over several segments, leading to activation of further trigger points along the spine. It is important to have these concepts in mind when palpating and assessing. Treatment should therefore address both the trigger points and articular dysfunction.

A radiculopathy model

Gunn's (1997a) theory states that chronic pain can occur in the event of:

- ongoing nociception or inflammation

- psychological factors such as a somatization disorder, depression or operant learning processes

- abnormal function in the nervous system.

According to Gunn, the myofascial pain syndrome can be the result of peripheral neuropathy, nerve root impingement and paraspinal muscle spasm. The spinal nerve dysfunction leads to an increase in muscle tone of the paraspinal muscles such as multifidi, leading to disc compression and irritation. This further irritates the neuropathy and a vicious cycle is created, one perpetuating the other. Which came first is a matter of discussion and debate. Gunn considers spondylosis, or bony/spur formation, as the most likely cause of nerve dysfunction. Gunn's treatment is aimed at the musculo-tendinous junctions or the location of the muscle motor points.

Gunn also considered that some of the deeper muscles of the back (for example, semispinalis thoracis, multifidus, rotatores muscles) must be palpated by needling, as they are beyond palpation by hand. He considered that only then can the affected muscle be identified and treated. Gunn (1997b, p.5) wisely uses 'the needle as a powerful diagnostic and treatment tool'. Gunn, when needling, is guided by the deqi response and tissue feedback. For example, Gunn describes the needling of fibrotic tissue as often being mistaken for bone and requiring a sustained force to penetrate. Needling should be an extension of palpation, as one can have a sense of the tissues being needled, tissue resistance, ease of needling, where the tip of the needle is, and the underlying structures and tissues being affected.

Chapman's points, TCM alarm and associated points

Osteopath Dr Frank Chapman in the 1930s showed a correlation between tender areas on palpation and associated visceral involvement. These tender areas are believed to be active neurolymphatic reflexes that can usually be palpated. The tenderness is usually in direct ratio to the chronicity and severity of the condition. For example, a group of reflexes are found between the spinous processes, where upon palpation the area feels spongy and has a close correspondence with the acupuncture points in the same location.

In TCM the same diagnostic reflexes exist where certain acupuncture points become sensitive to pressure when the meridian or organ to which they are reflexively connected is distressed. In a study by Kim (2007), an analysis of the similarity of locations between Chapman's neurolympathic reflex points and acupuncture points, the two systems identified anatomically 71.1 per cent of the anterior points and 93.1 per cent of the posterior points. When considering what one is feeling, a visceral reflex activity must be considered along with a musculoskeletal one.

Fascial considerations

Acupuncture meridians are believed to form a network throughout the body, connecting peripheral tissues to each other and to central viscera. Disruption of the meridian channel network is believed to be associated with disease, and needling of acupuncture points is thought to be a way to access and influence this system (Cheng 1987). Several authors have noted that interstitial connective tissue also fits this description, and conclusions have been drawn that acupuncture meridians tend to be located along fascial planes between muscles (Cheng 1987; Langevin and Jason 2002).

Thomas Myers, founder of Structural Integration (which has built upon the work of Ida Rolf), coined the term 'myofascial meridians', which are defined as anatomical lines that transmit strain and movement through the body's myofascia. These myofascial meridians were discovered through his analyses of human cadaver dissections that examined the interconnections of the body's fascia, tendons and ligaments, which form anatomical grids postulated as integral to the support and function of the locomotor system (Dorsher 2009). Myers (2009, p.237) himself comments on the close relationship between acupuncture meridians and the myofascial meridians: '…the close relationship between the two is inescapable, especially in light of recent research on and through the extracellular matrix.'

Broadly speaking, myofascial meridians present a mechanical stress model of fascia compared with the TCM model, which is visceral somatic. Trigger points tend to occur along myofascial meridians due to the way the body dissipates force along the course of these linkages (Neil-Asher 2014). Sharkey (2008) suggested a number of kinetic chains describing how the body moves by transmission of forces along these chains. This provides a more global view on movement. Janda (2012) always stated that compensations within chains create more dysfunctional movement, which is frequently seen in practice. Treatment may be over several sessions until the primary dysfunction is revealed and resolved. When considering the evidence, the suggested optimal treatment of any presenting MSK disorder must include the assessment and treatment of these myofascial meridians along with localized treatment for a truly successful outcome. Knowledge of the acupuncture meridians or myofascial meridians will enhance treatment outcome. Tender sites are almost consistently found in muscle at motor points or at muscle–tendon junctions (Gunn and Milbrandt 1976).

When considering where to needle, Langevin and Jason (2002, p.7) propose an enhanced effect at traditional points: '…the enhanced needle grasp response at acupuncture points may be due to the needle coming into contact with more connective tissue (subcutaneous plus deeper fascia) at those points.'

Needle grasp is not unique to acupuncture points but rather is enhanced at those points, so some knowledge of traditional acupuncture points may be useful. Palpate around the area of these points for the most effective treatment, using the palpation techniques as described earlier. Whilst needling, anywhere will have some effect, but needling at traditional points will have a better outcome due to the convergence of connective tissue that permeates the entire body (Langevin and Jason 2002).

If you consider just a handful of points such as Gallbladder 34, Triple Burner 15 and Bladder 10, these all have multiple muscles overlaying these points and have converging layers of fascia.

The fascia yet may reveal more secrets about visceral dysfunction. The technique of channel palpation involves palpating along the pathways of the 12 main acupuncture channels as an aid to diagnosis in TCM. Diagnostic palpation is particularly useful in the areas below the elbows and knees. Channel palpation provides a reliable, verifiable and relatively measurable way for practitioners to confirm diagnostic hypotheses derived from more mainstream Chinese medical approaches. Furthermore, because channel palpation provides significant information about the state of organ function, it can help focus diagnosis and treatment (Wang and Robertson 2007). It is beyond the scope of this book to describe fully the palpation process, but rather just to illustrate interpretations of fascia within TCM.

Conclusion

There are clearly many different ways of palpating, and even more different interpretations and possible treatments. This chapter is by no means the definitive guide on the subject, but we hope that it has encouraged the reader to engage and explore the process of palpation. As Denmei (2003, p.23) eloquently states: 'Satisfactory results can only be obtained when the four steps of diagnosis, point selection, point location and needles insertion all come together.'

References

Aubin, A., Gagnon, K., and Morin, C. (2014) 'A proposal to improve palpation skills.' *International Journal of Osteopathic Medicine 17*, 66–72.

Chaitow, L., Chaitow, S., Chemlik, S., Lowe, W., Myers, T., and Seffinger, M. (2010) *Palpation and Assessment Skills: Assessment through Touch* (third edition). Edinburgh: Churchill Livingstone.

Cheng, X. (1987) *Chinese Acupuncture and Moxibustion.* Beijing: Foreign Language Press.

Denmei, S. (2003) *Finding Effective Acupuncture Points.* Seattle, WA: Eastland Press.

Dorsher, P. (2009) 'Myofascial meridians as anatomical evidence of acupuncture channels.' *Medical Acupuncture 21*, 2.

Dowling, D. (1998) 'S.T.A.R.: a more viable alternative description system for somatic dysfunction.' *AAO Journal 8*, 2, 34–37.

Finando, S., and Finando, D. (2005) *Trigger Point Therapy for Myofascial Pain: The Practice of Informed Touch.* Rochester, VT: Healing Arts Press.

Gunn, C.C. (1997a) 'Myofascial pain, a radiculopathy model.' *Journal of Musculoskeletal Pain 5*, 4, 119–134.

Gunn, C.C. (1997b) *Intramuscular Stimulation (IMS) – The Technique.* iSTOP – Institute for the Study and Treatment of Pain. Available at www.istop.org/papers/imspaper.pdf, accessed on 23 July 2015.

Gunn, C.C., and Milbrandt, W.E. (1976) 'Tenderness at motor points: a diagnostic and prognostic aid for low-back injury.' *J. Bone Joint Surg. Am. 58*, 6, 815–825.

Janda, V. (2012) *The Janda Approach to Chronic Syndromes.* Available at www.jandaapproach.com/2012/11/02/timeless-vladimir-janda-quotes-and-concepts, accessed on 17 August 2015.

Kim, O. (2007) 'Comparative Analysis of the Topographical Locations of Acupuncture Points and Chapman's Reflex Points.' Unpublished thesis submitted in partial fulfilment of the degree of Master of Osteopathy, Unitec New Zealand, New Zealand. Available at http://unitec.researchbank.ac.nz/handle/10652/1347, accessed on 23 July 2015.

Langevin, H., and Jason, A. (2002) 'Relationship of acupuncture points and meridians to connective tissue planes.' *The Anatomical Record 269*, 6, 257–265.

Legge, D. (2011) *Close to the Bone: The Treatment of Painful Musculoskeletal Disorders with Acupuncture and Other Forms of Chinese Medicine* (third edition). Taos, NM: Redwing Book Co.

MacPherson, H. (1994) 'Body palpation and diagnosis.' *Journal of Chinese Medicine 44*, 5–12.

Mann, F. (2000) *Reinventing Acupuncture: A New Concept of Ancient Medicine* (second edition). Oxford: Butterworth-Heinemann.

Myers, T. (2009) *Anatomy Trains* (second edition). Edinburgh: Churchill Livingstone.

Neil-Asher, S. (2014) *The Concise Book of Trigger Points* (third edition). Chichester: Lotus Publishing.

Sharkey, J. (2008) *The Concise Book of Neuromuscular Therapy: A Trigger Point Manual.* Chichester: Lotus Publishing.

Travell, J.G., and Simons, D.G. (1999) *Myofascial Pain and Dysfunction: Upper Half of Body Volume 1: The Trigger Point Manual* (second edition). Baltimore: Lippincott Williams & Wilkins.

Wang, J.-Y., and Robertson, J. (2007) 'Channel palpation.' *Journal of Chinese Medicine 83*, 18–24.

Chapter 9

Deqi

There is a distinct cross-over between dry needling/Western acupuncture and traditional acupuncture techniques, so it is vitally important that we understand the original theories and how they relate to current modern thinking.

Our current concept of the mechanisms of action within dry needling is that in one aspect we are treating myofascial pain through the identification and needling of myofascial trigger points (MTrPs), and as an effect of acupuncture on a muscle we can evoke a local twitch response (LTR) – a spasm or contraction within the muscle – and this stimulates a pain-relieving effect among other responses.

This LTR has been referred to for centuries within traditional acupuncture techniques from all over the world. It is known as *deqi*, and is a fundamental aspect of traditional acupuncture treatments.

Deqi is usually translated as 'to obtain or grasp the qi when needling an acupuncture point'. The deqi sensation is felt by both practitioner and patient. Langevin, Churchill and Cipolla (2001) define deqi as a sensory component perceived by the patient together with a biomechanical component perceived by the practitioner.

There is a long-held belief that deqi is important in order to achieve positive therapeutic outcomes in acupuncture. However, it is unclear whether this is actually the case, as some acupuncture styles pay no clinical importance to it.

In one study of 574 members of the British Acupuncture Council (the primary organization of traditional acupuncturists in the UK), 87 per cent aimed to attain deqi (MacPherson *et al.* 2001). In a study of Chinese acupuncture patients, the majority of patients endorsed the importance of deqi in acupuncture therapy and 68 per cent further believed that the stronger the deqi sensation, the more effective the acupuncture treatment (Mao *et al.* 2007). Eighty-nine per cent of subjects reported that the needling sensation travelled away from the puncturing points or travelled among the needling points (MacPherson *et al.* 2001). Some authors suggest that Chinese-trained practitioners apparently perceive that Western patients react faster and to less stimulation than Chinese patients. Again there is disagreement as to whether deqi should be obtained if using electroacupuncture, as the stimulation is provided by the response to the electroacupuncture itself (see Chapter 12).

Essentially, as a practitioner, you are looking for deqi as feedback during the needling process, and adjusting your needle technique as a result of this feedback to elicit deqi. It is therefore important that the patient is aware of and understands deqi so as to guide and aid the practitioner.

Deqi as experienced by the patient is variously described as dull, aching, heavy, numb, radiating, spreading and tingling. The sensation of once having experienced deqi is unmistakable and is an unusual experience. Experiencing deqi as the practitioner is described as a fish biting a hook, needle grasp or a twitch response; these are generally attributed to the mechanical behaviour of the soft tissues surrounding/contracting around the needle. There may well be visible signs of deqi, including the twitch response, muscle tension, trembling, twitching, spasm and fasciculation. There may be redness around the needle insertion site indicating release of neuropeptides. Incorrect needling or missing the point has been described in classical texts as needling into a void, presumably describing the lack of feedback via the soft tissues and needle grasp.

Deqi is a complex phenomenon and may be influenced by a variety of factors. Patients may be inaccurate in reporting needle sensations as they wish to avoid further needling. They may not communicate accurately (or have the vocabulary for) what they are experiencing. Deqi is a subjective experience and is influenced by many factors, such as the constitution of a patient, severity of the illness, location of the acupuncture points and the needling techniques (Lundeberg 2013). Patients vary enormously in their response to acupuncture treatment: some will be extremely strong reactors, making their response greater to fewer needles, and so will need less treatment; whereas some patients will feel very little with lots of needles and lots of needle manipulation. In addition, each acupuncture treatment will include different points which will be needled at different depths with or without manipulation to produce differing results. The patient will also have a limit to the sensations that they can identify, especially when considering the possible number of acupuncture points used in a treatment.

Some practical suggestions

The practice of acupuncture is a diverse one, and when it comes to acupuncture needling there is no wrong or right way of doing it (as long as it is safe), as it is an individualized practice. The following are some suggestions based on observations and experiences that you may find helpful in your acupuncture practice.

Prior to commencing acupuncture, a description of the possible sensations produced by needling (deqi) must be accurately described to the patient. In patients with myofascial pain, the strong possibility of reproducing their symptoms must be described. Ideally, patients must be able to distinguish between deqi and pain. Communicate with the patient during needling and ask for clarification on the sensations felt by the patient. Some patients will struggle to communicate effectively, and in these cases it is best to ask simple, well-defined questions such as 'Is it reproducing your pain?' or 'Does it feel dull and achy?' to aid feedback as to whether or not deqi has been obtained.

Thicker needles are generally thought to produce deqi more easily, whereas needle grasp is less likely to happen when using smaller gauge needles that are highly polished, such as Japanese needles. However, with time and practice the same results can be generated with minimal discomfort to the patient (White, Cummings and Filshie 2008).

During needling it is extremely important that the practitioner focuses all of their attention on the needle, as needle grasp will be felt via the needle, which is essentially a very fine piece of metal. Again, when using very fine well-polished needles, this can be extremely subtle, but with time and practice it will become second nature and more intuitive.

Although it would be quite unacceptable to attempt most forms of treatment without defining the dose, acupuncture has so far remained without any means of quantification (Marcus 1994). For this reason, for the first few treatments it would be advisable to needle a few points and monitor the patient's reaction. This approach also has the benefit that future acupuncture treatments can be repeated using the same points or modified accordingly depending on the response. It is far better to needle a few points with precision and purpose and proceed with some caution, as opposed to blanket-bombing the patient with multiple needles.

Deqi may occur at any depth when needling. This may vary from shallow to deep, and sometimes a variety of needle depths are used during treatment to produce a variety of deqi responses (Nugent-Head 2013). If no deqi has occurred, needle manipulation may be used, including rotation, lift and thrust, flicking and twirling, to stimulate it. Again, the intensity of deqi is variable: it may last for a few seconds, it may slowly occur, it may suddenly occur or it may last for one minute or 20 minutes. Before any needle manipulation, it is worth trying some very fine adjustments, as these can suddenly produce dramatic deqi in patients. If sharp, shooting sensations are felt by a patient, then the possibility that the needle has been inserted directly into a nerve must be considered and withdrawal of the needle must be done immediately.

When needling, look for visible signs of deqi as described, but also monitor other visible clues to the patient's response such as rate of breathing, clenched fists, curled toes and sweating.

Mechanisms of action

It is widely thought that the mechanical deformation of sensory nerves (both myelinated and unmyelinated) in skin and muscle is responsible for the deqi sensation. Deqi can be a rich sensory experience and one that is stimulated by multiple nerve fibres (Wang *et al.* 1985). The main sensory nerves and possible relationship to acupuncture sensations are:

- Type II: numbness

- Type III: heaviness, distension, aching

- Type IV: soreness.

Some Western medical practitioners have proposed that deqi is simply an indication that the correct nerves have been stimulated (White *et al.* 2008). However, this does not explain the more subtle needling in some styles of Japanese acupuncture.

Langevin *et al.* (2001) argue that needle grasp is not due to muscle contraction but involves connective tissue. The authors demonstrated that needle rotation strengthens the mechanical bond between needle and connective tissue, which deforms the connective tissue surrounding the needle, delivering a mechanical signal into the tissue (possibly by deforming the sensory nerves). Increasing mechanical stresses by needle rotation surrounding connective tissue activates sensory receptors away from the site of needle insertion, possibly explaining sensations away from the needle site.

Interestingly, Langevin *et al.* (2001) demonstrated that lift and thrust techniques, which are commonly used in practice, result in a gradual build-up of torque at the needle–tissue interface. This perhaps explains why this technique is more tolerable for patients. Langevin *et al.* also proposed that acupuncture points may serve as a guide to where manipulation of the needle can result in a greater mechanical stimulus.

Langevin *et al.* (2001) further hypothesized that deqi causes acupuncture-induced actin polymerization in connective tissue fibroblasts, which may cause these fibroblasts to contract, causing further pulling of collagen fibres and a 'wave' of contraction and cell activation through connective tissue.

Sandberg *et al.* (2003) showed that deep needling with deqi (at GB-21, Upper Trapezius) in healthy subjects produced the most amount of blood flow. The same study suggested that the intensity of stimulation should be taken into consideration when treating chronic pain conditions, as the data suggested that there was no significant increase in blood flow with deqi when needling the patients with fibromyalgia.

The evidence so far...

Bovey (2006, p.27) states: 'There is no evidence as yet that any given type of acupuncture is better or worse than any other. Indeed, there are virtually no data at all comparing the clinical effects of different approaches.' At present we know that acupuncture works through a variety of different mechanisms, but different styles of acupuncture have yet to be clinically evaluated. As manual therapists we would never treat two patients the same; perhaps we would use the same techniques, but would adapt them accordingly to each patient. The same is true of acupuncture. With experience and intuition, greater clarity will emerge as to the appropriate dosage when needling different patients. For the practitioner, awareness of the different possibilities and variables when needling patients is important so as not to be alarmed when encountering differing responses.

References

Bovey, M. (2006) 'Deqi.' *Journal of Chinese Medicine 81*, 18–29.

Langevin, H.M., Churchill, D.L., and Cipolla, M.J. (2001) 'Mechanical signalling through connective tissue: a mechanism for the therapeutic effect of acupuncture.' *FASEB J. 15*, 2275–2282.

Lundeberg, T. (2013) 'To be or not to be: the needling sensation (de qi) in acupuncture.' *Acupunct. Med. 31*, 129–131.

MacPherson, H., Thomas, K., Walters, S., and Fitter, M. (2001) 'A prospective survey of adverse events and treatment reactions following 34,000 consultations with professional acupuncturists.' *Acupunct. Med. 19*, 2, 93–102.

Mao, J.J., Farrar, J.T., Armstrong, K., Donahue, A., Ngo, J., and Bowman, M.A. (2007) 'De qi: Chinese acupuncture patients' experiences and beliefs regarding acupuncture needling sensation – an exploratory survey.' *Acupunct. Med. 25*, 4, 158–165.

Marcus, P. (1994) 'Towards a dose of acupuncture.' *Acupunct. Med. 12*, 78–82.

Nugent-Head, A. (2013) 'Ashi points in clinical practice.' *Journal of Chinese Medicine 101*, 5–12.

Sandberg, M., Lundeberg, T., Lindberg, L.G., and Gerdle, B. (2003) 'Effects of acupuncture on skin and muscle blood flow in healthy subjects.' *Eur. J. Appl. Physiol. 90*, 1–2, 114–119.

Wang, K.M., Yao, S.M., Xian, Y.L., and Hou, Z.L. (1985) 'A study on the receptive field of acupoints and the relationship between characteristics of needling sensation and groups of afferent fibres.' *Evid. Based Complement. Alternat. Med. 2013*, 483105. Online. Available at www.ncbi.nlm.nih.gov/pmc/articles/PMC3766991, accessed on 23 July 2015.

White, A., Cummings, M., and Filshie, J. (2008) *An Introduction to Western Medical Acupuncture.* Edinburgh: Churchill Livingstone.

Chapter 10

Planning Treatment

Treatment strength and the patient's sensitivity

There is no golden rule for using or incorporating dry needling/medical acupuncture into your treatment protocol, and patients new to acupuncture techniques will respond very differently. As such, each patient and treatment is to be taken on its own merit and adjusted accordingly.

It is advised that 'less is more' with new patients, and therapists should avoid over-stimulating in the first few sessions, by which we would advise that new patients are treated with fewer needles, and those needles are not overly stimulated until the patient's tolerance and how the patient reacts to treatment has been established.

Not everyone will respond to the use of dry needling, and with patients that show no response to treatment after several sessions, then the use of electroacupuncture would be appropriate as a way of increasing the strength and effectiveness of the technique.

Treatment duration

In terms of needle duration, it has been seen that acute conditions respond to short needling times, whereas chronic conditions respond to longer duration. That being said, treatment can last anywhere from inserting and immediately removing the needles, to leaving the needles in for up to 30 minutes. Patients should not be left alone during the treatment, and tolerance and sensitivity should be verbally monitored to ensure patient comfort.

Acupuncture before, during or after manual therapy?

This will be down to the judgement of the therapist. There is no strict rule that acupuncture must only be used before soft tissue work or manipulation, for example – it simply doesn't work like that. Treatment needs to be individualized to the specific patient, and the therapist may wish to use acupuncture techniques before, during or after other therapeutic modalities. The only considerations are to ensure that the skin is clean and clear of lotions or oils, all the needles have been fully removed before other therapeutic modalities are employed, the patient is not bleeding and you have followed the safety guidelines already stipulated.

Step-by-step guide

Before starting treatment, ensure that:

- you have all your equipment ready and to hand

- the patient is in a comfortable position

- the skin is clean and clear of oils or lotions

- a case history has been fully completed and the patient's previous sensitivities and treatment reactions have been noted

- new patients have been informed of possible treatment reactions, and have a clear understanding that they can stop the treatment at any point if it becomes uncomfortable

- the area being worked on is clear and free of clothing.

The following is relevant during the treatment:

- Locate and palpate the point of pain within the muscle, identify any risk factors or neurovascular structures to be aware of before needling, and ensure that you use the correct grip of the target muscle.

- Choose the correct needle insertion technique for the muscle: perpendicular, oblique or inferior techniques depending on anatomical structures around the site.

- Choose your style of handling the needle and insert it into the target muscle.

- Check patient comfort, and then stimulate the needle to elicit a twitch response. Ensure you are aware of the treatment time for needle retention depending on whether the condition is chronic or acute.

- Once the treatment has finished, remove all the needles and place them into a sharps bin, and inform the patient that all the needles have been removed.

- Check for any bleeding, and give appropriate aftercare advice.

- Note down any immediate treatment reactions, whether good or bad.

Part IV

NEEDLING TECHNIQUES

Chapter 11

Muscles

Techniques and Clinical Implications

Supraspinatus

Palpation: Sitting within the supraspinatus fossa, the supraspinatus runs along and underneath the acromion, attaching onto the greater tubercle of the humerus. Palpate the spine of the scapula as your landmark and move upwards into the fossa; the fibres of the supraspinatus run parallel to the spine.

Pain referral pattern: The supraspinatus will primarily refer pain to the anterior portion of the shoulder and to the lateral epicondyle region; there are secondary referral sites in the posterior shoulder and upper arm.

Needling technique: With the patient prone, palpate for areas of pain. The needle should be inserted near the supraspinatus fossa towards the bulk of the muscle with the direction in a longitudinal plane, aiming towards the greater tubercle of the humerus.

Adaptations: The patient should ideally be prone or side lying. Needle length between 1 inch and 1.5 inches.

Clinical implications: This technique, whether used with the patient prone or side lying, will take the needle towards the front of the scapula, and expose the risk of passing into the intercostal space and towards the pleural cavity.

The lung in a thin person lies 0.5–1 inch under the skin and there is the danger of pneumothorax if the needle is inserted too deeply. It is advised to use perpendicular needling techniques for areas close to the lungs, and in some cases it is also advised to grasp the muscle and pick it up to reduce the risks further.

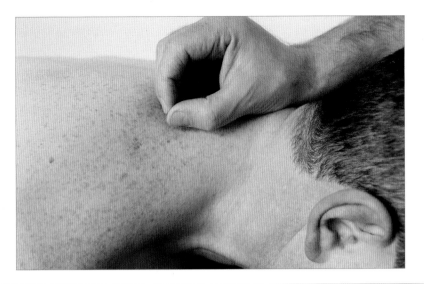

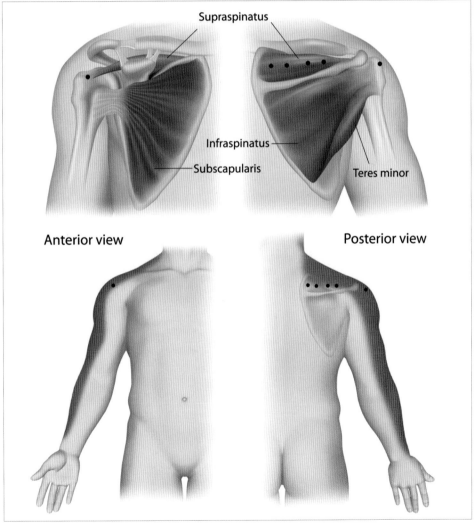

Figure 11.1 Supraspinatus trigger points

Infraspinatus

Palpation: The infraspinatus sits within the infraspinatus fossa, with the bulk of the muscle being superficial to palpate; its insertion is on the greater tubercle of the humerus. Palpate the spine of the scapula as your landmark and move downwards into the infraspinatus fossa; the fibres run laterally towards the greater tubercle of the humerus and sit underneath the bulk of the deltoid.

Pain referral pattern: The infraspinatus will primarily refer pain to the anterior portion of the shoulder and to the area of the mid-thoracic, the medial border of the scapula. There are secondary points in the cervical spine and, more often, in the anterior portion of the arm, forearm and into the thumb.

Needling technique: Palpate the infraspinatus and highlight any areas of pain. The needle will be placed directly into that point within the muscle belly in a perpendicular direction towards the scapula.

Adaptations: The patient should ideally be prone or side lying. Needle length between 1 inch and 1.5 inches.

Clinical implications: Due to its location sitting above the bulk of the scapula, as long as there is no compromise within the scapula allowing the needle to penetrate through, there are no clinical implications.

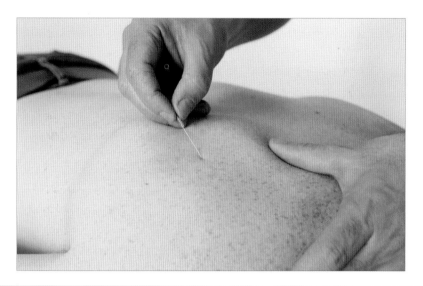

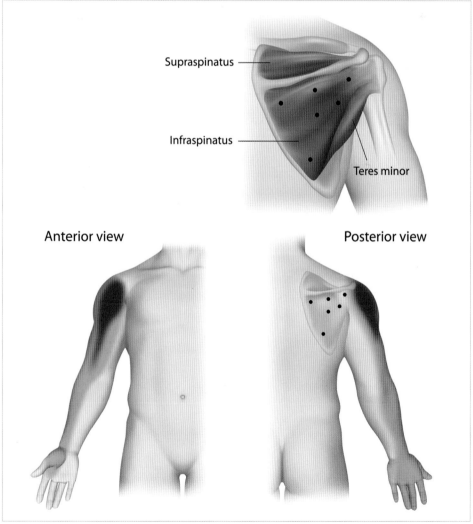

Supraspinatus

Infraspinatus

Teres minor

Anterior view

Posterior view

Figure 11.2 Infraspinatus trigger points

Deltoid

Palpation: The deltoid sits in a triangle shape at the top of the shoulder, split into three sections: the anterior, medial and posterior fibres of the muscle. The three heads of the deltoid all originate from the lateral one third of the clavicle, acromion and spine of scapula. Insert into the deltoid tuberosity, which is also the same insertion point for the trapezius.

Pain referral pattern: The deltoid will primarily refer pain very locally, to the anterior and posterior shoulder girdle. There are secondary sites in the anterior and posterior forearm.

Needling technique: Ideally sit the patient upright; then you can needle all the sections of the muscle from the anterior, medial and posterior. If this is not possible, then you will need to move the patient from supine to needle the anterior and medial, and to prone to affect the posterior muscle. Due to the location and muscle bulk, you can needle directly into any areas of pain that are highlighted.

Adaptations: You may need to use needles from 1 inch to 2 inches depending on the musculature of the patient.

Clinical implications: None.

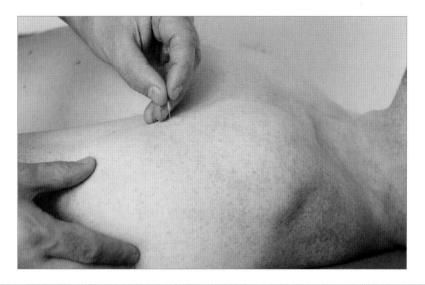

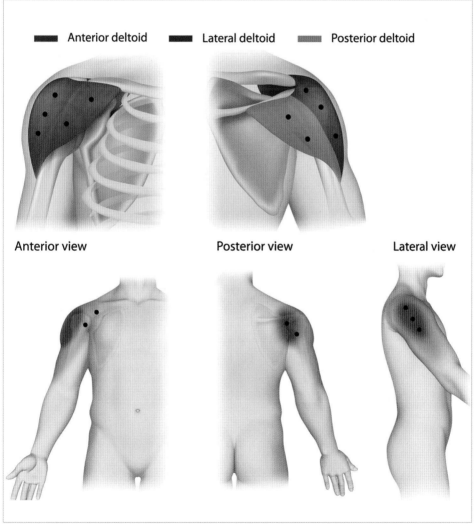

Figure 11.3 Deltoid trigger points

Subscapularis

Palpation: The subscapularis sits within the subscapular fossa and inserts into the lesser tubercle of the humerus and the front of the capsule of the shoulder joint.

Pain referral pattern: The subscapularis will refer pain very locally around the location of the muscle. It has also been shown to primarily refer pain into the carpal tunnel area of the forearm.

Needling technique: To gain access to the bulk of the muscle, have the patient supine, place the arm above the patient's head to expose the muscle bulk and use a perpendicular needling technique.

Adaptations: Patient should ideally be prone or supine. Needle length between 2 inches and 3 inches.

Clinical implications: This technique, whether used with the patient prone or supine, will take the needle behind the scapula, and expose the risk of passing into the intercostal space and towards the pleural cavity.

The lung in a thin person lies 0.5–1 inch under the skin and there is the danger of pneumothorax if the needle is inserted too deeply. It is advised to use shallow needling techniques for areas close to the lungs, and in some cases it is also advised to grasp the muscle and pick it up to reduce the risks further.

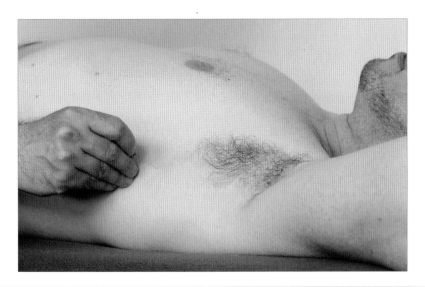

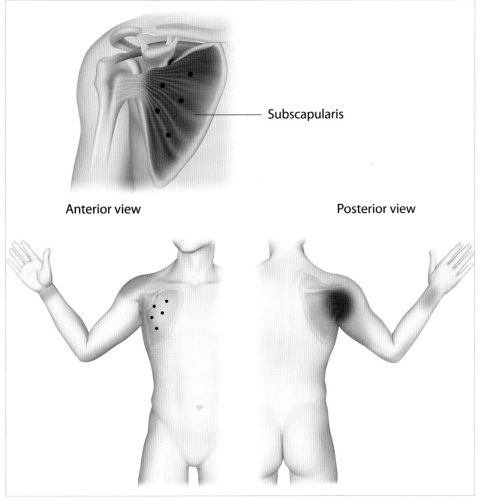

Subscapularis

Anterior view

Posterior view

Figure 11.4 Subscapularis trigger points

Teres minor

Palpation: The teres is a small muscle situated between the lateral border of the scapula, inserting into the greater tubercle of the humerus. It sits between teres major and the infraspinatus. The muscle is small and can be quite difficult to grasp.

Pain referral pattern: Localized pain referral into the upper back, shoulder and arm.

Needling technique: With the patient prone, drop the arm off the couch and work from the border of the scapula as your landmark. Move laterally off the lateral border and you will slide onto the teres minor. To confirm your location, ask the patient to laterally rotate the shoulder and the teres minor will contract. Grasp the muscle with your thumb and forefinger, bring the muscle slightly away from the rib cage, and the needling insertion will be lateral and towards the abdomen.

Adaptations: The patient should ideally be prone or side lying. Needle length between 1 inch and 1.5 inches.

Clinical implications: By grasping the muscle and bringing it away from the rib cage, you reduce the risk of compromising that area. The needle direction is always away from the rib cage. There are no clinical implications.

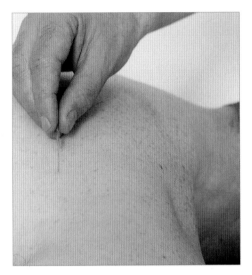 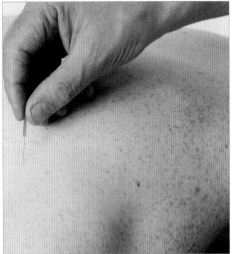

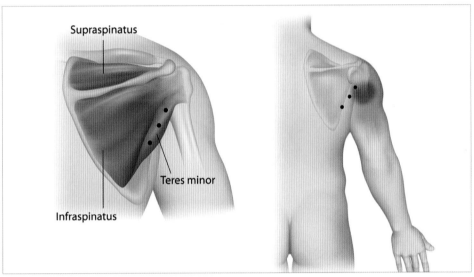

Supraspinatus

Teres minor

Infraspinatus

Figure 11.5 Teres minor trigger points

Latissimus dorsi and teres major

Palpation: The latissimus dorsi is one of the largest muscles within the back and sometimes the most overlooked within manual therapy. It is closely linked with the teres major, originating from the spinous processes of the last six thoracic vertebrae, the lower four ribs and the posterior iliac crest. This muscle spans along the back, inserting into the crest of the lesser tubercle of the humerus. The teres major has its origin on the inferior side of the lateral border of the scapula and it too inserts into the crest of the lesser tubercle of the humerus.

Pain referral pattern: The latissimus dorsi refers locally into the mid-thoracic spine and secondarily into the posterior aspect of the arm and shoulder; the teres major, which is very closely associated, also refers primarily into the posterior arm and shoulder.

Needling technique: *Latissimus dorsi.* With the patient prone, start at the lowest portion to affect the inferior fibres nearest the lower four ribs. Grasp the muscle between the thumb and forefinger and bring it away from the chest wall. The needle will be placed directly into the muscle belly, towards the couch, lateral to the chest wall. Repeat this action and make your way up the latissimus dorsi, needling the medial and superior fibres to affect the whole muscle.

Needling technique: *Teres major.* With the patient prone, using the same grasping techniques, work up the latissimus dorsi and move medially towards the lateral border of the scapula. On that lateral border will be the teres major, and the needle is inserted directly into the muscle or laterally and inferiorly towards the scapula.

Clinical implications: The patient may respond strongly to needling of the latissimus dorsi, and a strong local twitch response may be felt as you needle the length of the muscle. By gripping the muscle and pulling it away from the chest wall, you minimize any risk of penetrating the chest wall.

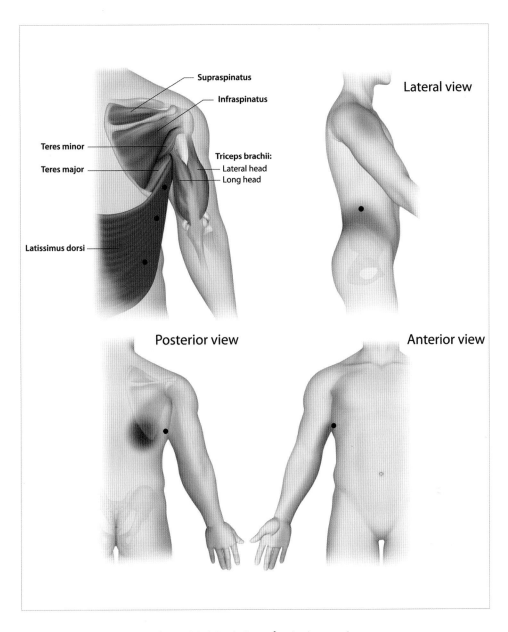

Supraspinatus

Infraspinatus

Teres minor

Teres major

Triceps brachii:
Lateral head
Long head

Latissimus dorsi

Lateral view

Posterior view

Anterior view

Figure 11.6 Latissimus dorsi trigger points

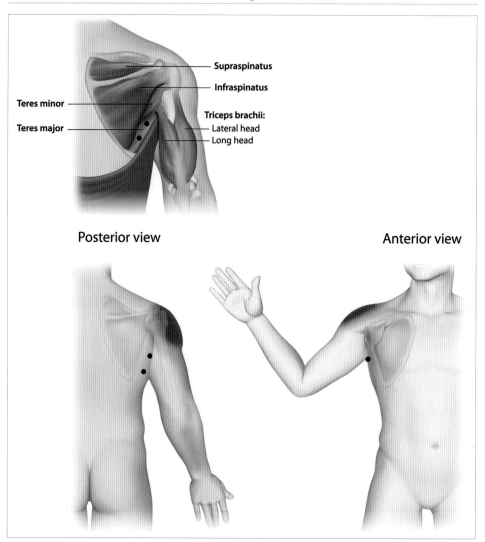

Figure 11.7 Teres major trigger points

Rectus femoris

Palpation: The rectus femoris is one of four parts of the quadriceps femoris group of muscles that extend the leg at the knee joint, and is located between the tensor fasciae latae and sartorius. The rectus femoris helps to flex the thigh and also anteriorly tilts the pelvis, at the hip joint. With the patient in supine position, with thighs on the table and legs hanging off, stand to the side and palpate on the anterior surface, close to the hip. Externally rotate the hip and resist flexion. Support with a hand on the distal leg, close to the ankle joint, to provide resistance. Locate the rectus femoris via the proximal tendon of the tensor fasciae latae or sartorius. Extend the leg and feel for the contraction of the muscle and continue palpating distally.

Pain referral pattern: Pain is referred to the front and centre of the knee and can cause problems fully flexing the knee and/or extending the hip.

Needling technique: With the patient in a supine position, use a perpendicular angle into the bulk of the muscle, or into specific spots of pain within the muscle itself.

Clinical implications: There are no clinical implications within the rectus femoris. The femoral artery lies very deep underneath the muscle, so if using much longer needles such as 2 or 3 inches then caution should be applied.

Vastus medialis, vastus intermedius and vastus lateralis

Palpation: The vastus medialis, vastus intermedius and vastus lateralis make up three of the four subcomponents of the quadriceps femoris. The three muscles contribute to the extension of the knee. The quadriceps forms a trilaminar tendon insertion at the patella, and the vastus medialis and vastus lateralis form an intermediate layer. The vastus intermedius makes up the deep layer. Palpate whilst seated, with flexed knee and thigh maintained in horizontal position. Stabilize and palpate the vastus medialis of the distal medial thigh. Due to the depth of the muscle, to access the vastus intermedius lift the rectus and palpate from the medial or lateral side.

Pain referral pattern: The quadriceps femoris muscle group, which includes the vastus medialis, vastus intermedius and vastus lateralis, is responsible for the referred pain to the front and inner side of the knee and to the mid-thigh area. Vastus medialis can also refer deep pain to the knee joint.

Needling technique: This group of muscles is needled in the same technique. With the patient supine, identify the target muscle and needle perpendicularly into the muscle or directly into any painful spots within the muscle itself.

Clinical implications: None.

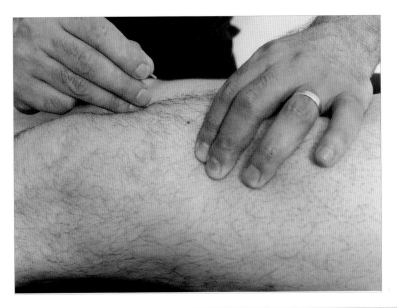

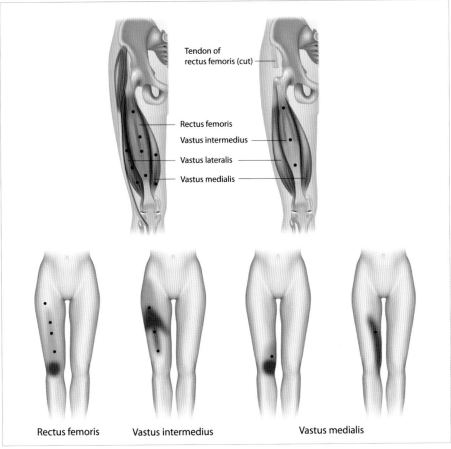

Figure 11.8 Quadriceps muscle trigger points

Pectoralis minor

Palpation: Situated next to the rib cage and running perpendicular, the pectoralis minor has its origins on the third, fourth and fifth ribs. Insert onto the coracoid process of the scapula. Due to its location, several major structures run underneath the pectoralis minor: the brachial plexus, axillary artery and vein.

Pain referral pattern: The pectoralis minor will refer pain locally and into the anterior portion of the chest and shoulder.

Needling technique: With the patient supine, and with the arm slightly abducted, palpate the lateral edge of the pectoralis major, and as you slide underneath this muscle you are able to access the pectoralis minor. The needle should be inserted in an inferior/shallow depth above the rib cage, and the needle should be pulsed laterally towards the coracoid process. As with the latissimus dorsi, an alternative method is to pinch the muscle and raise it up from the rib cage.

Adaptations: Patient should ideally be supine or side lying. Needle length between 1 inch and 1.5 inches.

Clinical implications: When needling the pectoralis minor, care should be taken not to needle into the intercostal space or penetrate the rib cage – an inferior needling technique is recommended for this area. Avoid deep needling, being aware of the structures which are situated below the muscle and the potential for neurovascular compression by this muscle.

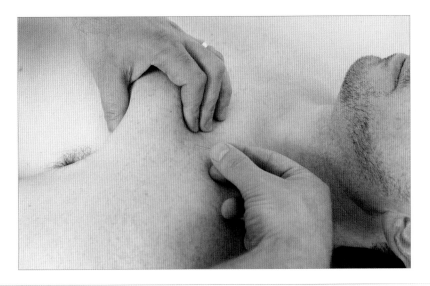

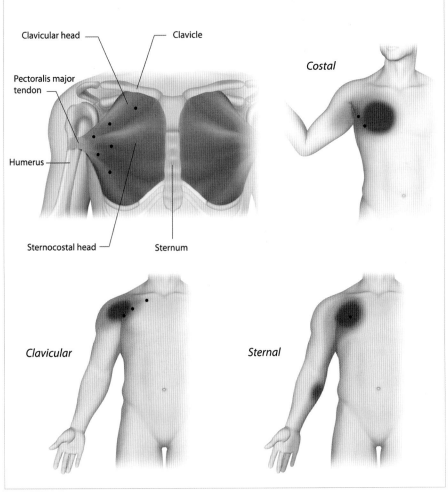

Clavicular head — Clavicle

Costal

Pectoralis major
tendon —

Humerus —

Sternocostal head — Sternum

Clavicular

Sternal

Figure 11.9 Pectoralis major trigger points

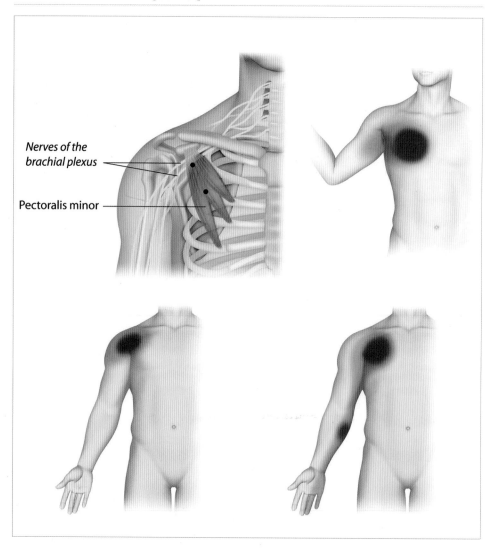

Figure 11.10 Pectoralis minor trigger points

Coracobrachialis

Palpation: This small yet important muscle is situated deep in the arm. Its origins are at the coracoid process of the scapula and it inserts into the mid-shaft of the humerus. To palpate the coracobrachialis, get the patient to lay supine, and abduct and laterally rotate the shoulder. As you palpate the medial side of the arm towards the armpit, get the patient to gently adduct the arm horizontally and the coracobrachialis will contract.

Pain referral pattern: The coracobrachialis will refer pain locally and into the anterior portion of the shoulder and posterior aspect of the arm.

Needling technique: The patient should be lying in a supine position, with the medial portion of the upper arm exposed by abducting and laterally rotating the shoulder. The needle is inserted directly into the muscle belly near to the coracoid process.

Clinical implications: This area may be sensitive to bruising, and its close proximity to the neurovascular bundle of the upper arm should be considered when needling. Avoid the brachial artery.

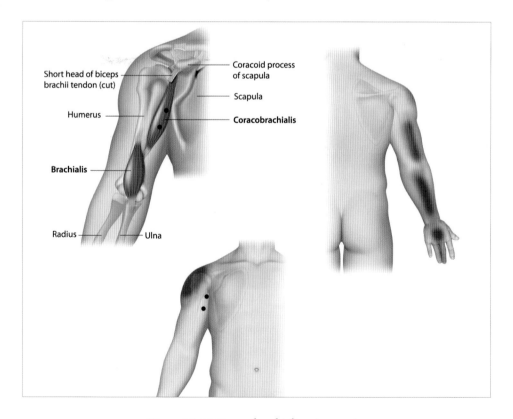

Figure 11.11 Coracobrachialis trigger points

Biceps brachii

Palpation: The biceps brachii is located on the anterior border of the humerus. This thick muscle belly has two origins: the short head of the bicep originates in the coracoid process, and the long head is situated close by in the supraglenoid tubercle. As these two heads merge, insert into the tuberosity of the radius and the aponeurosis of the biceps brachii.

Pain referral pattern: The biceps brachii will refer pain locally and into the anterior portion of the shoulder and arm.

Needling technique: With the patient supine, grip the bicep and pick up the muscle slightly, allowing you to accurately palpate any areas of pain. The needle should be inserted laterally; this avoids the neurovascular bundle on the medial/inner arm.

Adaptations: The patient should ideally be supine or side lying. Needle length between 1 inch and 1.5 inches.

Clinical implications: Limited. If the application of the needle is from the lateral aspect, avoiding the medial part of the muscle, you reduce any risk of compromising the radial nerve or affecting the neurovascular bundle. Avoid the brachial artery.

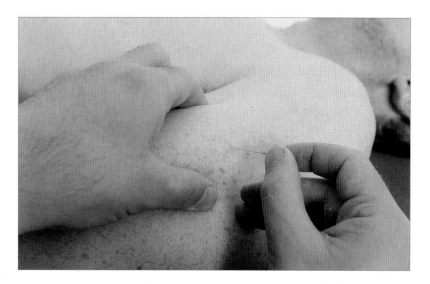

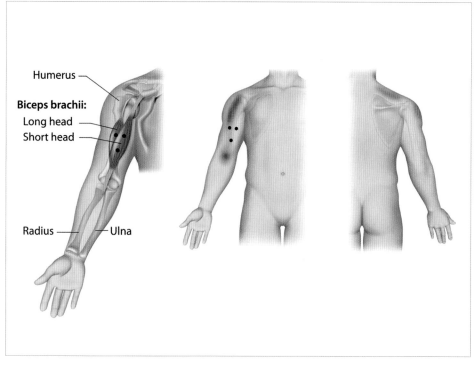

Figure 11.12 Biceps brachii trigger points

Triceps

Palpation: Made up of three heads, this muscle is the only one situated on the posterior arm. It is superficial and easy to palpate and needle. The origins of the long head are at the inferior tubercle of the scapula, the lateral head is on the proximal half of the humerus, and the medial head is on the posterior surface of the distal half of the humerus. These three heads insert into the olecranon process.

Pain referral pattern: The triceps can refer primarily locally and to the front of the arm. Also, it has a secondary referral to the medial and lateral epicondyle and olecranon.

Needling technique: With the patient prone, palpate the muscle for any areas of pain, and the needle insertion will be directly into any highlighted trigger points.

Adaptations: The patient should ideally be prone or side lying. Needle length between 1 inch and 1.5 inches.

Clinical implications: None.

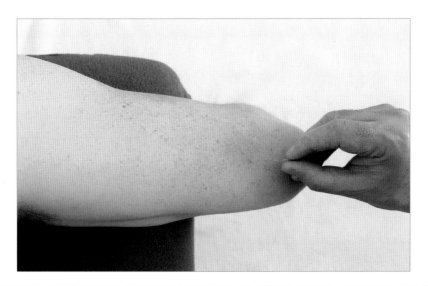

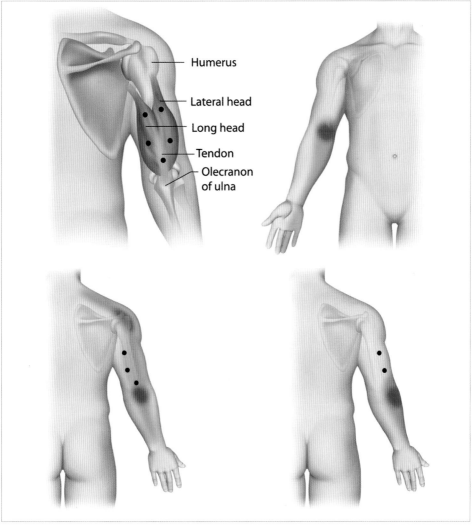

Humerus

Lateral head

Long head

Tendon

Olecranon
of ulna

Figure 11.13 Triceps trigger points

Masseter

Palpation: Situated between the zygomatic arch and the angle and ramus of the mandible, the masseter is a thick, powerful band of muscle that is easily palpated between these two points. To confirm, ask the patient to gently bite down, tensing the jaw muscles and allowing the masseter to rise up.

Pain referral pattern: The masseter will refer to the cheek and jaw on the affected side and into the temporomandibular joint, causing pain.

Needling technique: With the patient either supine or side lying, locate the masseter muscle, ensure the patient is relaxed and insert the needle directly into the muscle at a perpendicular angle.

Clinical implications: The therapist should be aware of needle length and needle depth when needling this muscle group. Avoid needling too deeply in case the needle punctures the inside of the mouth.

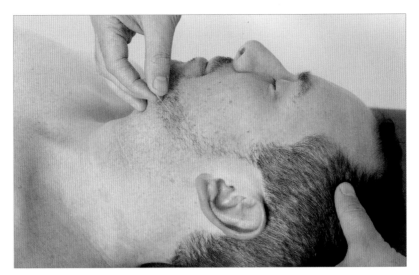

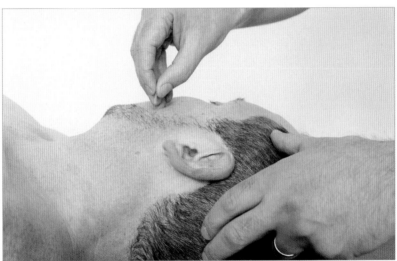

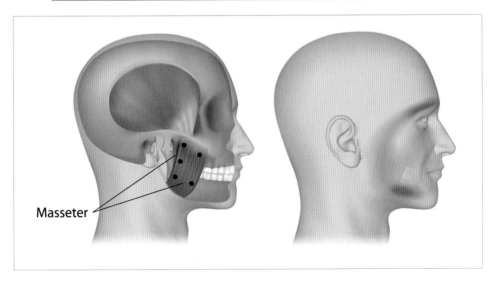

Masseter

Figure 11.14 Masseter trigger points

Temporalis

Palpation: Located roughly an inch superiorly above the zygomatic arch and stretching out to the temporal fossa and fascia, the temporalis muscle spans a thick muscular band. Reconfirm the location by asking the patient to gently bite down and the muscle will contract.

Pain referral pattern: The temporalis can refer pain into the eyebrow and temple area on the affected side, and into the temporomandibular joint.

Needling technique: The muscle can be needled in two different ways. Ensure the patient is either supine or side lying, and either use an inferior needle technique to thread the needle towards the temporal fossa, or perpendicularly into the bulk of the muscle.

Clinical implications: Locate the superficial temporal artery first, and avoid needling directly into that, as any bleeding can cause large bruising around that area.

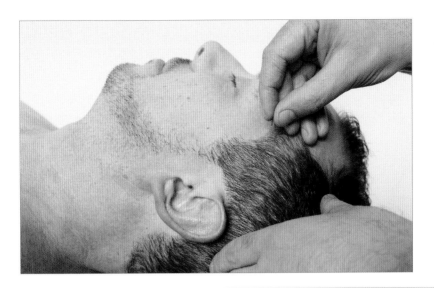

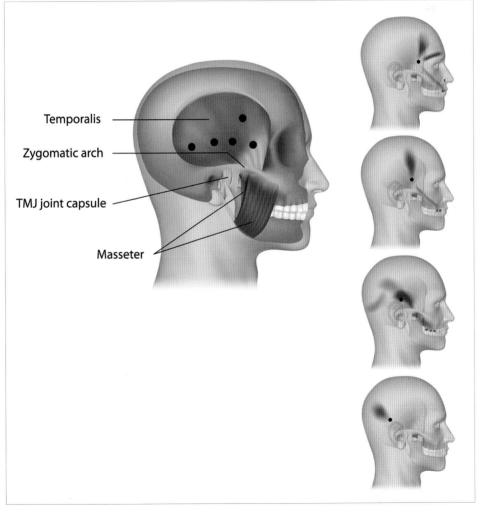

Figure 11.15 Temporalis trigger points

Upper trapezius

Palpation: This is one of the most commonly treated muscle groups within manual therapy and an area where most people can feel pain and discomfort. It stretches from as far up as the occipital protuberance across to the clavicle and acromion process and down to the level of T12. The trapezium is easily located as the fibres form the bulk of muscle sitting across the top of the shoulders bilaterally. Grasp the trapezius muscles and bring them slightly superiorly away from the bony structures.

Pain referral pattern: This large muscle can refer to a number of places, primarily into the posterior head and neck, temporomandibular joint and into the mid-thoracic spine, but also into the posterior aspect of the shoulder.

Needling technique: Perpendicular needling into the bulk of the muscle is the safest technique for this area. However, be aware of the apex of the lung. When using longer needles, do not use an inferior needling technique. The handle of the needle should never point towards the pelvis.

Adaptations: Depending on the size of the patient, use a 1–1.5 inch needle into this area. The patient should be aware that the trapezium muscles can respond strongly to acupuncture in this area and a strong local twitch response can be felt.

Clinical implications: This technique, whether used with the patient prone or side lying, will take the needle towards the front of the scapula, and expose the risk of passing into the intercostal space and towards the pleural cavity.

The lung in a thin person lies 0.5–1 inch under the skin and there is the danger of pneumothorax if the needle is inserted too deeply. It is advised to use shallow needling techniques for areas close to the lungs, and in some cases it is also advised to grasp the muscle and pick it up to reduce the risks further.

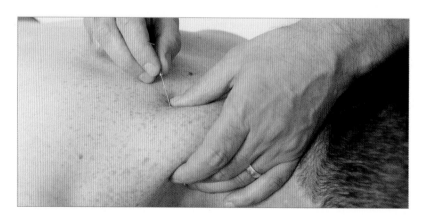

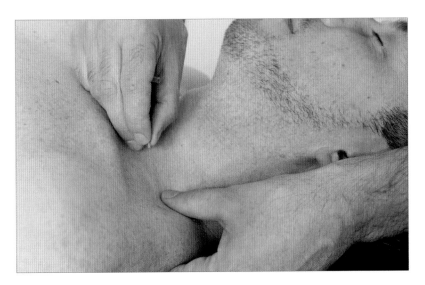

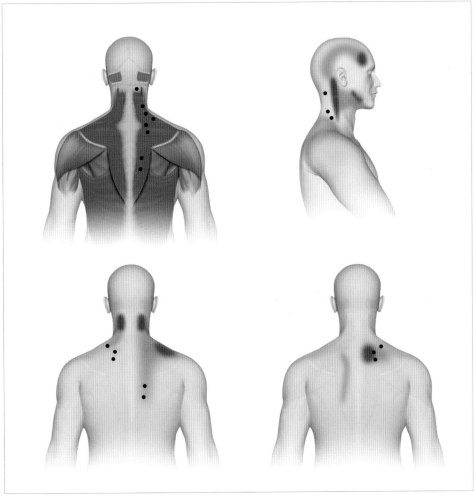

Figure 11.16 Upper trapezius trigger points

Levator scapula

Palpation: Work through the upper fibres of the trapezius in order to palpate the levator scapula muscle. The levator scapula spans from the medial border of the scapula to the transverse processes of the upper cervical spine (C1–C4). To accurately locate the muscle, locate the superior medial border of the scapula and drop off that superior angle. Palpate the levator muscle fibres as they angle laterally towards the cervical spine.

Pain referral pattern: The levator scapula will refer pain locally over the bulk of the muscle, from the medial border of the scapula and mid-thoracic spine, and it will refer superiorly into the cervical spine.

Needling technique: With the patient either prone or side lying, locate the levator scapula and use a perpendicular angle of needle insertion into the muscle belly.

Clinical implications: As with muscle groups in the vicinity of the rib cage, it is crucial to avoid directing the needle towards the pleura of the lung. Use a perpendicular angle into the muscle bulk, and never angle the needle inferiorly towards the rib cage or pelvis in order to make sure the lung is avoided at all times.

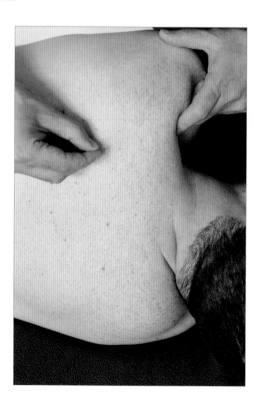

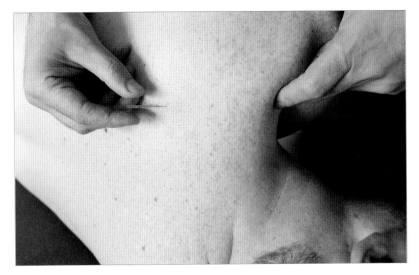

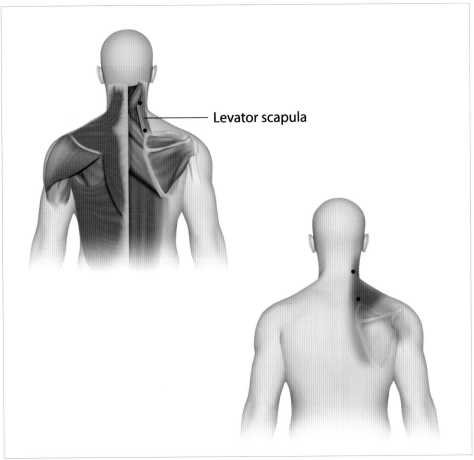

Figure 11.17 Levator scapula trigger points

Splenius capitis and cervicis

Palpation: The oblique fibres of the splenius muscles run deeply to the rhomboids and trapezius muscles in the upper back; they are difficult to palpate. The bony landmarks to work from at the origin of the muscle are the spinous processes of C7 to T6, and the fibres run to the transverse processes of the upper C spine and the superior nuchal line. The muscle runs close to the spine, and becomes easier to locate as you palpate the lamina groove of the cervical spine.

Pain referral pattern: This group refers into the posterior aspect of the head and neck, and to the top of the head and around the frontal and temporal areas of the face.

Needling technique: With the patient either prone or side lying, grasp the muscle; between the thumb and forefinger and lightly pull the muscle away from the bone. The needle should be inserted into the muscle at a lateral angle.

Clinical implications: Ensure that the needle is not angled towards the vertebral artery and that the depth of the needle is kept shallow to avoid invading into the cervical spine.

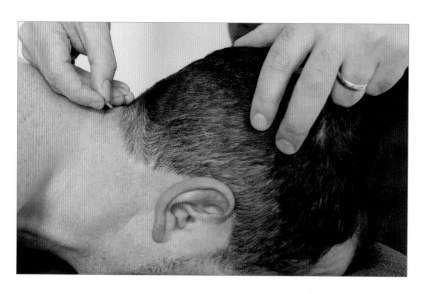

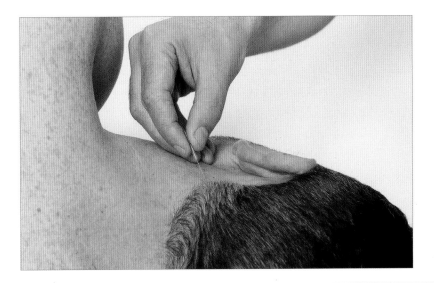

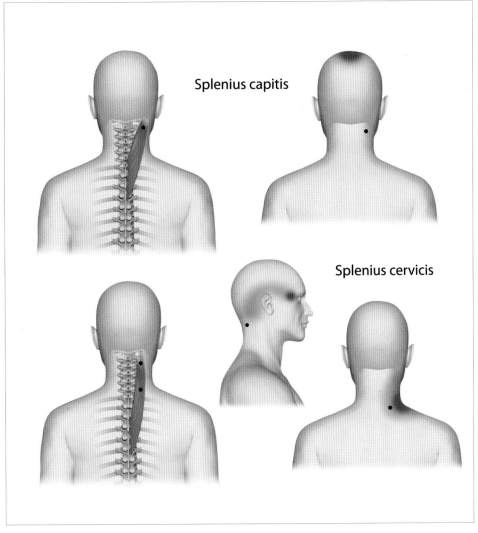

Figure 11.18 Splenius capitis and cervicis trigger points

Suboccipitals

Palpation: There are eight muscles that make up the suboccipitals and they are some of the deepest muscles in the superior cervical spine. They can be a contributing factor in chronic neck and head pain, and patients suffering with headaches. With the patient prone, locate the first palpable spinous process of C2, and the transverse process of C1, as the start point of the suboccipital muscle group. Trace out to the superior nuchal lines the outer portion of the suboccipitals.

Pain referral pattern: The referral pattern for the suboccipital muscles refers into the high cervical spine, and laterally around to the temple and eye brow.

Needling technique: The needle is inserted perpendicularly into the bulk of the muscle; the therapist should then angle the needle slightly and advance it in the direction of the patient's nose, in order to access the bulk of the muscles. Use four needles into this group and this will resemble a TCM technique called a 'peacock's tail': two needles bilaterally will be inserted laterally and inferiorly to the external occipital protuberance; the second two needles will then be inserted between those needles and the mastoid process.

Adaptations: 1 inch needles are advised to be used in this area.

Clinical implications: Although extremely uncommon and difficult to do with the length of the needles, you should be aware of the location of the vertebral artery and foramen magnum, and these structures are to be avoided.

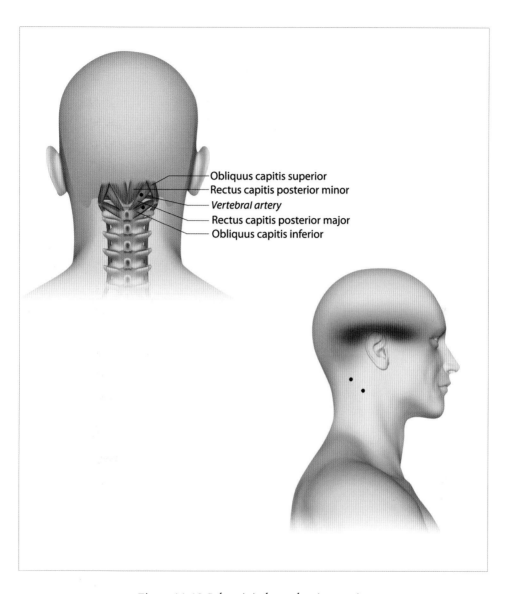

Figure 11.19 *Suboccipital muscle trigger points*

Sternocleidomastoid

Palpation: This thick portion of muscle can be found on the lateral portion of the neck, very superficially forming a large 'V' from the manubrium sterni and medial section of the clavicle and stretching up to the mastoid process of the temporal bone, at the superior nuchal line. It is a strong neck stabilizer and can be greatly affected in cases of whiplash.

Pain referral pattern: Pain can be felt locally, into the head and neck, and into the cheek and jaw.

Needling technique: The patient may be supine or side lying. Gently move the sternocleidomastoid away from the midline of the throat using a pincer grip with your non-needling hand. The angle of needle insertion is perpendicular to the table while supine, or perpendicular to you if the patient is side lying. You are able to needle the sternocleidomastoid mid-belly, at the sternal and clavicular attachment sites.

Clinical implications: The carotid artery is the main concern with this technique. The aim of lifting the sternocleidomastoid away from the midline of the throat is to move the sternocleidomastoid away from the carotid arteries and thus minimizing the risk of needling the carotid artery.

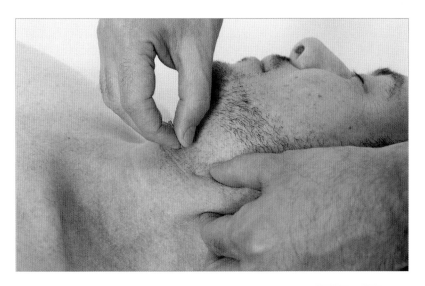

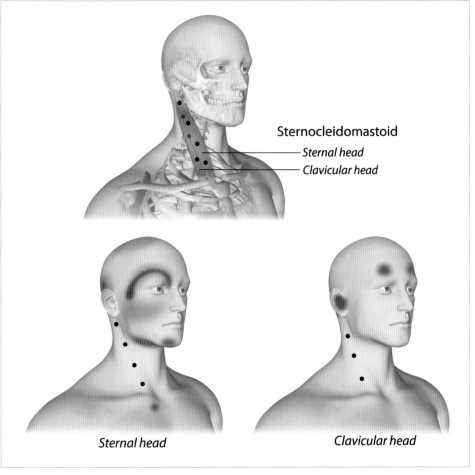

Figure 11.20 Sternocleidomastoid trigger points

Thoracic and lumbar multifidus

Palpation: These are deep spinal muscles which are an important contributor to thoracic and lumbar rotation, lateral flexion and extension. They originate from the posterior surface of the sacrum and articular processes of the lumbar vertebra and transverse processes of the thoracic spinous process. Insert into the spinous process 2–4 vertebrae higher than its origin.

Locate the spinous process of the target vertebrae and move an inch laterally to locate the transverse process. Between these two points lies the multifidus muscle.

Pain referral pattern: Locally around the spinous processes of the vertebra; lumbar, lower and mid-thoracic pain.

Needling technique: With the patient prone (ideally), or side lying if they are unable to lie prone, needle directly adjacent to the spinous process of the relevant area. You should be needling into the paravertebral gutter. The angle of the needle is approximately 30 degrees to the skin and is directed medially towards the vertebral lamina.

Clinical implications: In the thoracic spine you must not needle more than one finger width from the spinous process due to the risk of infiltrating the pleural space. In the lumbar spine there is no precaution of needling more than one finger width away from the spinous process.

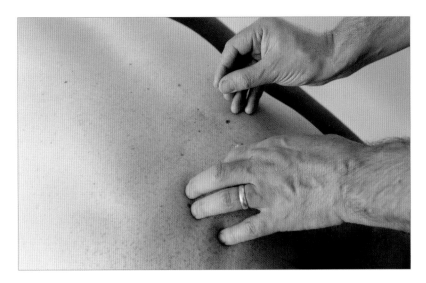

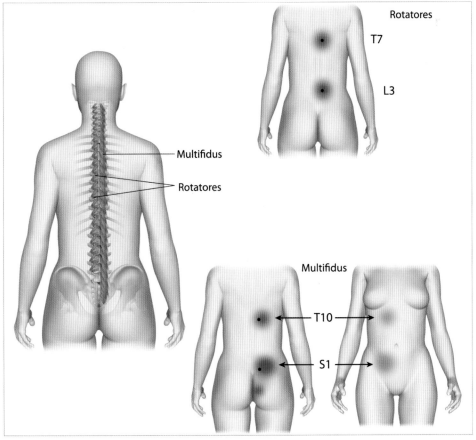

Figure 11.21 Multifidus and rotatores trigger points

Rhomboid major and minor

Palpation: Spanning from the medial border of the scapula onto the thoracic vertebrae at the levels of T2–T5, the rhomboid muscle is deep to the trapezius but is still considered as a superficial back muscle. With the patient prone, trace the medial border of the scapula towards the levels of T3–T5, asking the patient to place their hand behind their back, raising the scapula up. This can expose the muscle.

Pain referral pattern: Mid-thoracic back pain.

Needling technique: The patient can be prone or side lying. If needs must, then the patient could also be seated. While in the side-lying position, the patient's arm must be secured to avoid them moving. The main aim is to keep them in a comfortable position. The rhomboid muscles can be needled either towards their attachment sites or transverse to the fibres. This will depend on your palpation and how many fibres are affected.

Clinical implications: If needling transverse to the fibres, use the inferior needling technique. This will minimize the risk of infiltrating the pleural space and causing a pneumothorax. If needling towards the attachment, then using an angle of 30 degrees to the skin is advisable.

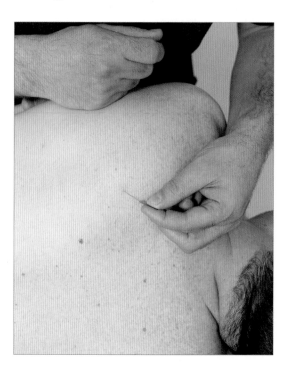

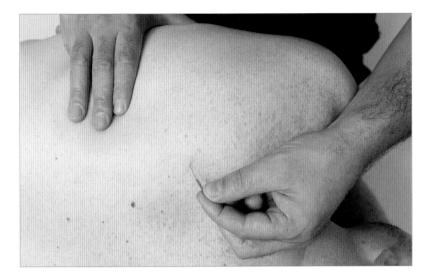

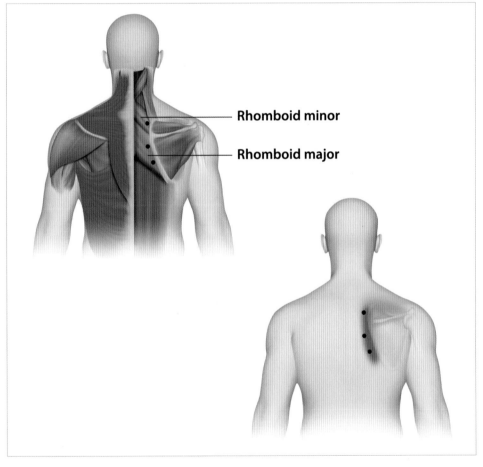

Figure 11.22 Rhomboid major and minor trigger points

Quadratus lumborum

Palpation: With deep and some superficial layers, the quadratus lumborum sits under the layers of the lumbar erector spinae muscles. This structure is a common contributor to lower back pain due to its connection to the spine and pelvis.

The muscle starts at the iliac crest and iliolumbar ligament, fanning up to the 12th rib and the transverse processes of the lumbar spine. As it is deep, it can be difficult to locate and palpate for acupuncture. With the patient prone, locate the spinous process of the lumbar spine and move laterally. Then move your fingers across the erector spinae muscles. The muscle will drop, allowing palpation towards the belly button at a 45-degree angle towards the quadratus lumborum.

Pain referral pattern: Lower back, iliosacral and gluteal pain.

Needling technique: The quadratus lumborum muscle can be needled in the prone or side-lying position. The needles will be placed between the iliac crest and the 12th rib. At the level of L4 (approximately) is the main window of opportunity to access the quadratus lumborum. The needle angle should aim towards the transverse process to achieve the correct depth and be angled towards the midline of the body or the umbilicus.

Clinical implications: The upper needle is angled towards the patient's contralateral posterior superior iliac spine and not inserted above the 12th rib. This is to avoid any risk of penetration of the kidney.

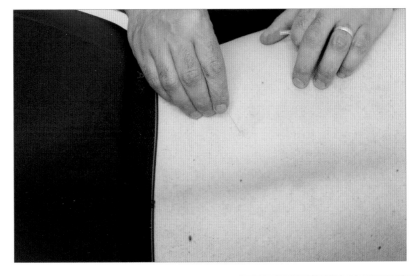

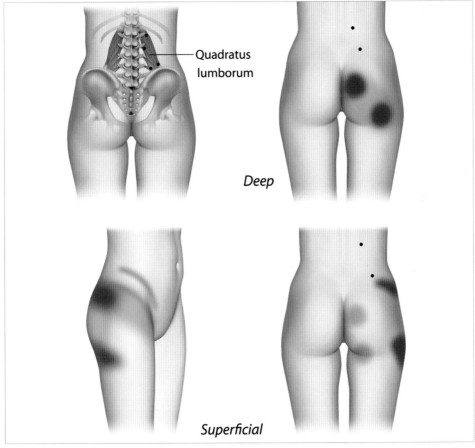

Figure 11.23 Quadratus lumborum trigger points

Cervical multifidus

Palpation: The cervical multifidus muscles insert onto the lower cervical facet capsular ligaments and the cervical facet joints. They are small, strong muscles that can be a direct source of pain in traumatic injuries such as whiplash where the head is thrown forwards and backwards at speed.

Pain referral pattern: Pain can be felt locally, into the head and neck, and into the cheek and jaw.

Needling technique: With the patient either prone or supine lying, insert the needle in a perpendicular direction to the skin, aiming between the articular processes between C4 and C7.

Precautions: When using this technique, it is advised that you avoid direct needling towards the spinous processes to avoid infiltration of the spinal canal.

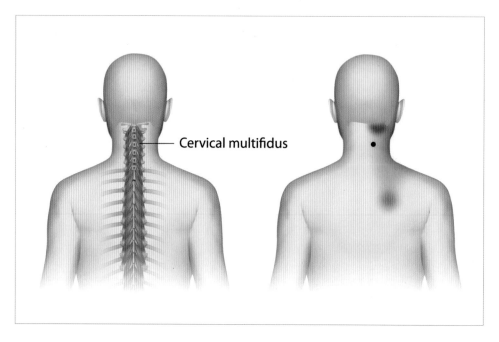

— Cervical multifidus

Figure 11.24 Cervical multifidus trigger point

Lumbar erector spinae

Palpation: The erector spinae is a large, thick superficial muscle that originates near the sacrum and extends vertically up the length of the thoracic spine. It lies bilaterally with the vertebral column and extends alongside the lumbar, thoracic and cervical sections of the spine.

Pain referral pattern: Pain can be felt locally to the site or can refer towards the sacroiliac joint on the same side of dysfunction and towards the glutes.

Needling technique: With the patient prone (ideally) or side lying, needle directly adjacent to the spinous process of the relevant area. You should be needling into the paravertebral gutter. The angle of the needle is approximately 30 degrees to the skin and is directed medially towards the vertebral lamina.

Clinical implications: In the thoracic spine you must not needle more than one finger width from the spinous process due to the risk of infiltrating the pleural space. In the lumbar spine this precaution is not needed.

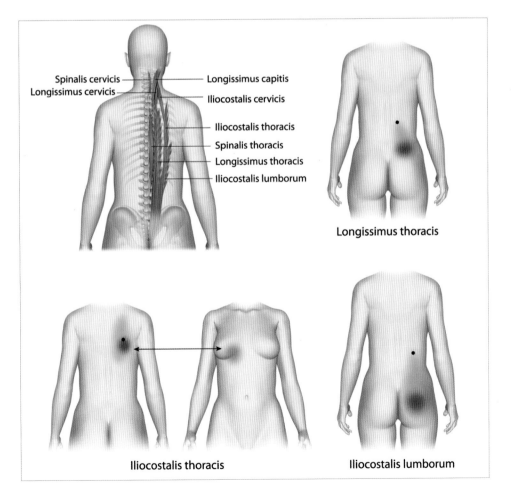

Figure 11.25 Lumbar erector spinae trigger points

Scalenes

Palpation: The scalenes are made up of three lateral vertebral muscles – the scalenus anterior muscle, scalenus medius and scalenus posterior – and pass up from the ribs into the sides of the neck. The muscles elevate the first rib to allow breathing and facilitate movement and rotation of the neck. The scalene muscles elevate the first two ribs when the muscles are fixed from above, and bend and flex the spinal column when working from below. The scalenes can be easily palpated seated or supine. Rotate the head and neck to the opposite side, at the spinal joints. Laterally flex the head and neck to the same side. Resist lateral flexion.

Pain referral pattern: Pain in the scalenes is variable and complex and is usually referred to other areas of the body. Pain spreads from the neck into the chest and upper back and through the arm to the hand, and can also trigger symptoms associated with sinuses, swallowing and hearing.

Needling technique: While the patient is supine, ask them to take a sharp intake of breath while palpating the area. This will enable you to locate the scalenes.

To access the anterior portion, you must locate the anterior triangle formed by the clavicular attachment of the sternocleidomastoid, the base of the clavicle and the jugular vein.

The direction of needling for the anterior scalene is perpendicular to the skin and approximately 1–1.5 inches above the clavicle. You must direct the needle towards the transverse process.

The middle scalene muscles are accessed through the triangle of the base of the clavicle, posterior scalene muscle and the brachial plexus. The direction of needling for the middle scalene is towards the posterior tubercle and transverse processes of the cervical spine.

Clinical implications: You must needle the scalenes 1–1.5 inches above the clavicle to minimize the risk of infiltrating the pleural space and impacting the apex of the lung.

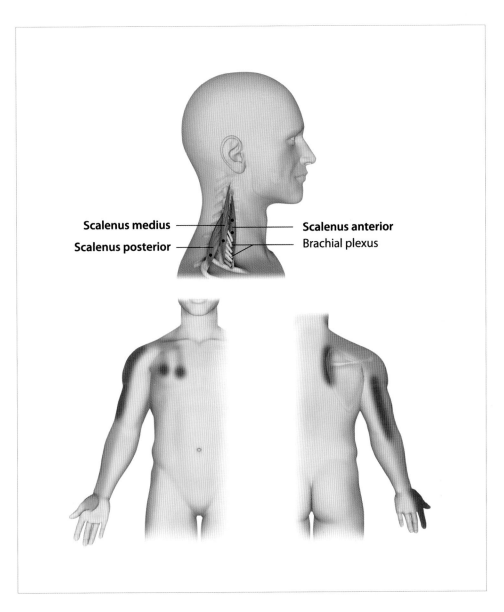

11.26 Scalene muscle trigger points

Wrist flexors – flexor carpi radialis, flexor carpi ulnaris, flexor digitorum superficialis, flexor digitorum profundus, flexor pollicis longus

Palpation: Flexors located in the forearm make up three layers of muscles – superficial, intermediate and deep – and are responsible for pronation and flexion of the wrist and fingers. The superficial layer contains the long bellies of the flexor carpi radialis, palmaris longus and flexor carpi ulnaris. The intermediate and deep layers contain the wide bellies of the flexor digitorum superficialis and flexor digitorum profundus, which can be felt from their origin. Sections of these muscles can be isolated for palpation. The radial hand on the anterior side flexes the hand at the wrist joint. Flex and abduct the wrist whilst assisting elbow flex. Flex the fingers. Roll over the tendons to feel the contraction of the flexors.

Pain referral pattern: Forearm flexors refer pain to the inside of the wrist, and are proximal to the sides of the thumb and little finger.

Needling technique: The patient ideally should lie supine with the forearm in the anatomical position. The needle is inserted perpendicular to the radius and ulna, depending on the muscle being treated.

Clinical implications: If the patient receives symptoms of irritation from the median and/or ulnar nerve and there is no ease in their symptoms, then remove the needle and avoid that precise location.

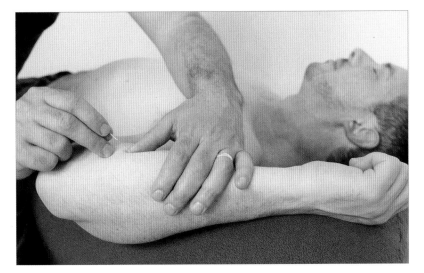

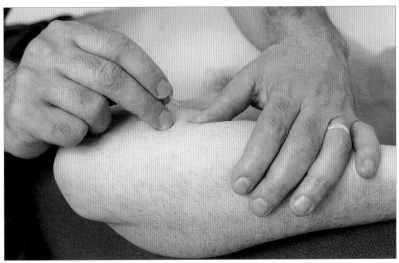

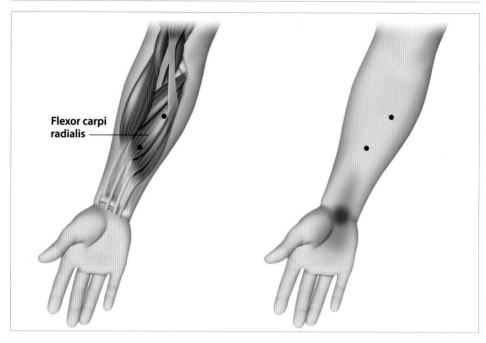

11.27 Flexor carpi radialis trigger points

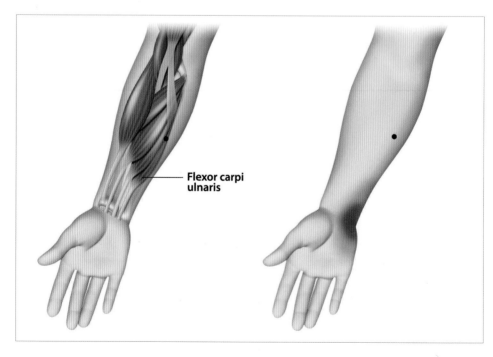

Figure 11.28 Flexor carpi ulnaris trigger point

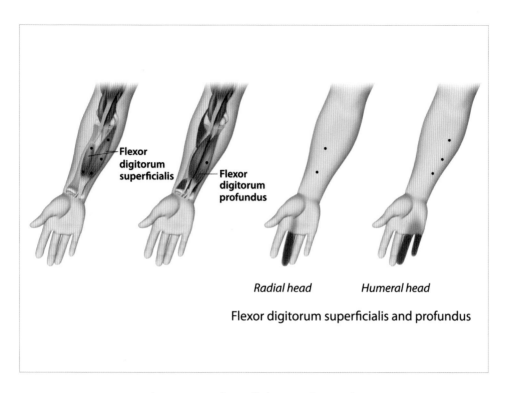

Figure 11.29 Flexor digitorum trigger points

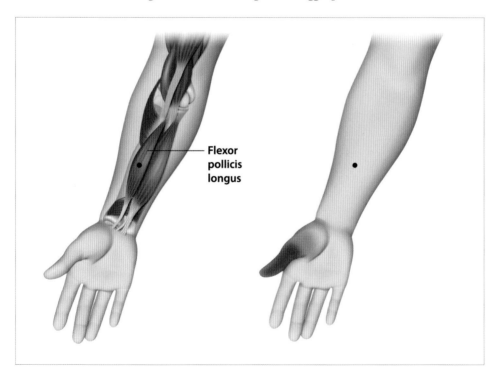

Figure 11.30 Flexor pollicis longus trigger point

Wrist extensors – extensor carpi radialis longus, extensor carpi radialis brevis, extensor carpi ulnaris and extensor digitorum

Palpation: There are four superficial muscle extensors in the hand and wrist that originate from the lateral side of the humerus. These muscles are smaller and more sinewy than the forearm flexors and are also more accessible. The extensor carpi radialis longus and extensor carpi radialis brevis are located on the posterior side of the brachioradialis. The extensor carpi ulnaris is situated alongside the ulna. Between these muscles lies the extensor digitorum. Palpate by flexing the elbow to locate the ulnar and brachioradialis, and then extend and relax the wrist. Explore the contraction of the sinewy muscles.

Pain referral pattern: The forearm extensors refer pain to the back of the wrist and also to the outside aspect of the wrist.

Needling technique: The patient ideally should lie supine with the forearm in the anatomical position. The needle is inserted perpendicular to the radius and ulna, depending on the muscle being treated.

Clinical implications: If the patient receives symptoms of irritation from the median and/or ulnar nerve and there is no ease in their symptoms, then remove the needle and avoid that precise location.

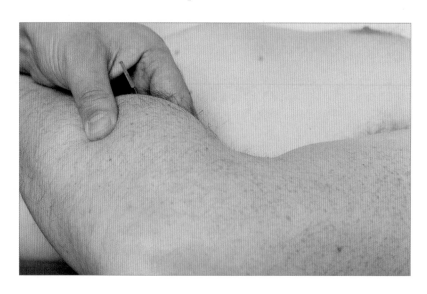

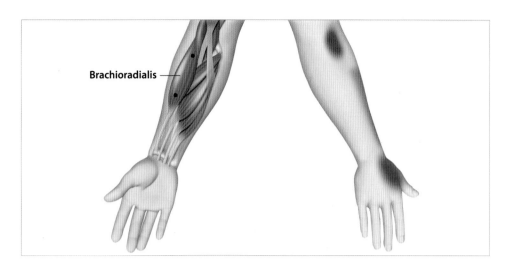

Figure 11.31 Brachioradialis trigger points

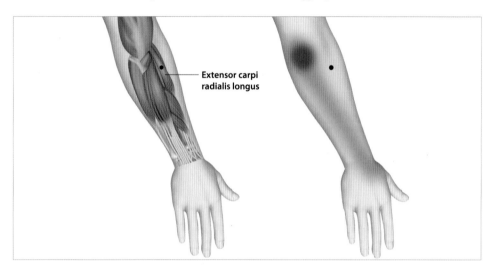

Figure 11.32 Extensor carpi radialis longus trigger point

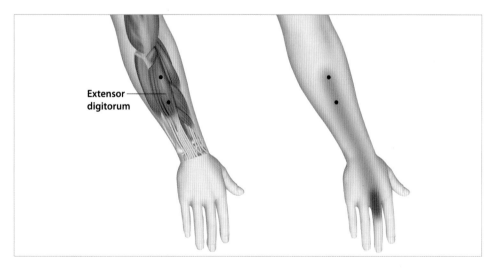

Figure 11.33 Extensor digitorum trigger points

Supinator

Palpation: The supinator is located in the upper forearm and is deeply concealed by superficial muscles. It originates from the inferior aspect of the lateral epicondyle of the humerus and the crest of the ulna. The flat supinator laterally wraps around the upper third of the radius and inserts into the posterior, anterior and lateral aspects. The muscle is responsible for the ordinary supinatory movements of the forearm. Fully flex the elbow to midpronate the forearm. The muscle can be palpated once the arm is supinated against resistance.

Pain referral pattern: Pain is referred locally and also into the wrist and the base of the thumb. The backside web between the thumb and index finger can also be affected. The supinator is primarily responsible for causing 'tennis elbow' and movement-and-rest pain in the outer elbow.

Needling technique: The supinator muscle can be needled with the patient supine or side lying. The non-needling hand uses a pincer grip to lift the extensors away from the radius. This allows access to the supinator muscle. Needling should be via the palmar side of the extensors.

Clinical implications: There is a small risk that you may irritate a superficial branch of the radial nerve. This may cause the patient moderate discomfort with some pins and needles but will not have a lasting effect.

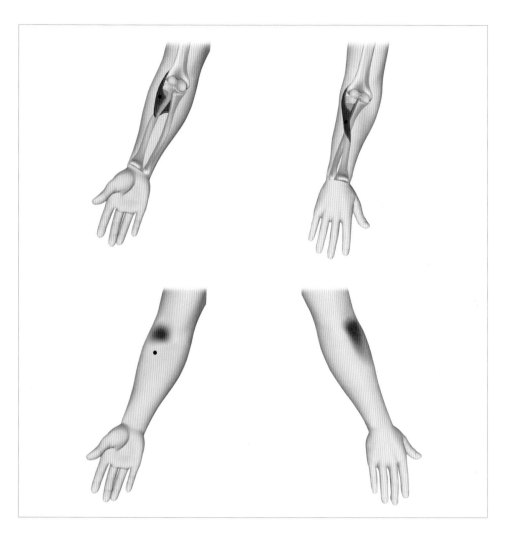

Figure 11.34 Supinator trigger point

Pronator teres

Palpation: The pronator teres is located between the inner elbow and the centre of the radius bone in the forearm and is the most lateral of the superficial flexor compartment muscles. The pronator teres passes laterally downwards and attaches via a flattened tendon. The muscle pronates the forearm and helps to flex the elbow. The pronator can be easily seen and palpated when the forearm is resisting pronation. The pronator quadratus initiates pronation of the forearm and lies within the flexor compartment. The inaccessible, fleshy, quadrangular-shaped muscle traverses the lower quarter of the anterior surface of the ulna to the anterior radius surface. Isolate the radial artery pulse and locate the anterior surface of the radius. Flex and pronate the wrist and use your thumbs to explore the tissue and small contractions.

Pain referral pattern: Pronator pain is referred locally, predominantly towards the base of the thumb.

Needling technique: The optimal position for this technique is the patient lying supine with the forearm in the supinated position. Needling of this muscle is to the proximal, medial portion, which is located slightly below the medial epicondyle.

Clinical implications: Needling should remain 0.5–1 inch below the medial epicondyle to avoid the median and ulnar nerves.

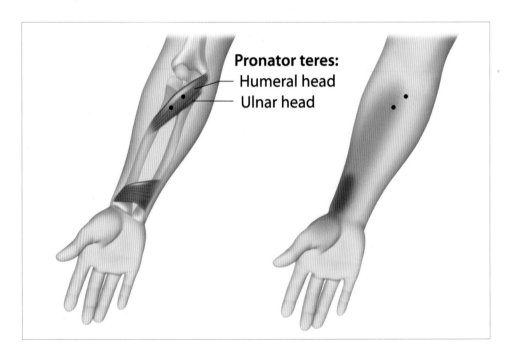

Pronator teres:
— Humeral head
— Ulnar head

Figure 11.35 Pronator teres trigger points

Serratus anterior

Palpation: The serratus anterior is a large muscle that is located between the scapula and thorax, with origins to the lateral ribs. The serratus anterior lies alongside the underside of the subscapularis and inserts on the undersurface of the scapula's medial border. From behind, locate the lateral border of the scapula. From the lateral edge palpate inferiorly using four fingers and work towards the ribs. Follow the section of the serratus to the origin. Flex the shoulder and elbow. Resist protraction of the scapula to ensure the correct location. The serratus posterior runs under the shoulder blade to the ribs. Palpating this muscle requires moving the shoulder blade out of the way by reaching the arm across the chest.

Pain referral pattern: Serratus anterior pain is typically referred to the side and lower part of the shoulder blade. Serratus posterior pain is primarily referred locally and can cause a deep pain under the shoulder blade. Pain can also be felt in the back of the shoulder, elbow, back of the upper arm and forearm and the little finger.

Needling technique: Locate the muscle and, using a pinching technique, grip the muscle and pull it slightly away from the intercostal space. Using an inferior needling technique, insert the needle at a perpendicular angle. Avoid angling the needle towards the lungs.

Clinical implications: Due to its anatomical location near to the lung space, ensure that you avoid needling towards the lungs at all times to ensure that the lung is not penetrated.

Gluteus maximus, gluteus medius and gluteus minimus

Palpation: Gluteus maximus, gluteus medius and gluteus minimus make up the gluteal group of muscles and, as their names suggest, range in size. Gluteus maximus is the largest and most posterior and originates at the posterior sacrum and ilium. The muscle extends the femur, at the hip, and laterally rotates the hip.

Palpate by extending and laterally rotating the thigh, at the hip. As the muscle contracts, palpate to discern the borders and tone.

Gluteus medius is partially superficial and located on the side of the hip. It originates at the ilium crest and contracts and stabilizes the pelvis. Abduct the thigh at the hip and feel for the contraction of muscle fibres. Use your thumbs to palpate the fleshy area. Gluteus minimus is inaccessible and originates on the posterior ilium. This muscle works with the gluteus medius during rotation and abduction of the femur at the hip.

Pain referral pattern: The glutes primarily refer pain to the lower back and locally to the gluteal region. Gluteus minimus has a very large and complex distribution of referred pain and can affect the tensor fascia latae, hamstrings, quadriceps, gastrocnemius and peroneal muscle groups. The most common referred pain pattern is known as side sciatica.

Needling technique: The patient may be prone or side lying. The depth of the needle will be dependent on the anatomy and the amount of adipose tissue. As the gluteus maximus is the most superficial gluteal muscle, then the depth of needle may not need to be substantial.

Clinical implications: If you irritate the sciatic or superior gluteal nerves and the patient's response does not ease, then remove the needle and possibly insert a new needle in a slightly different location.

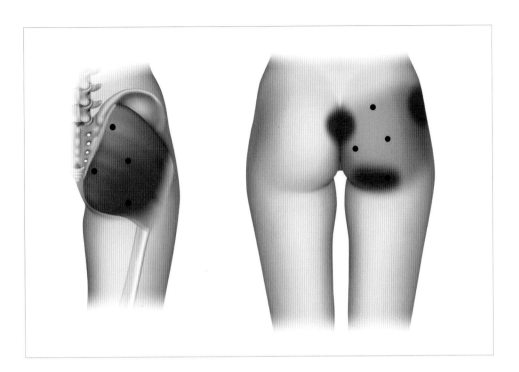

Figure 11.36 Gluteus maximus trigger points

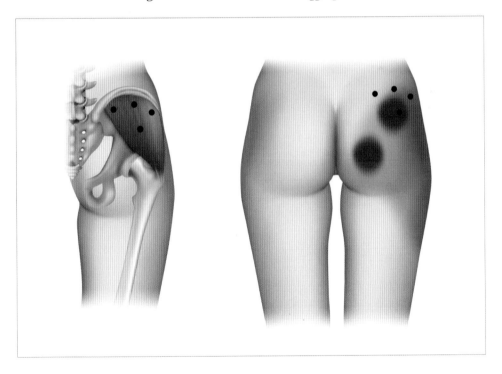

Figure 11.37 Gluteus medius trigger points

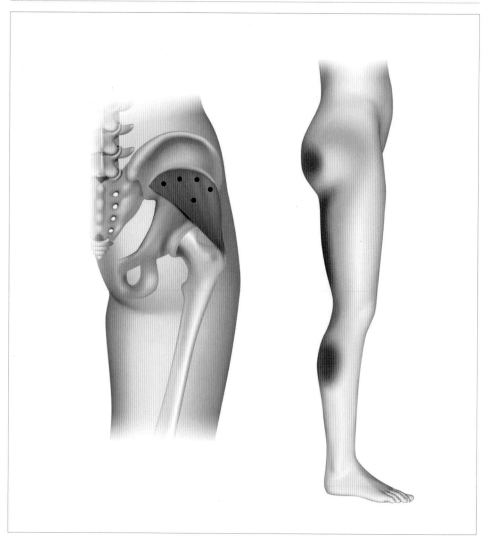

Figure 11.38 Gluteus minimus trigger points

Obturator

Palpation: The obturator internus and obturator extermus form part of the six muscles that make up the deep lateral rotator group, located in the pelvis. The muscles work together to rotate the thigh at the hip and to contralaterally rotate the pelvis. The obturator extermus is covered by the large quadratus femoris and is therefore not visible. To palpate, start from the prone position, with the leg flexed at the knee joint. Place your fingers halfway between the posterior superior iliac spine and sacrum apex. Rotate the thigh at the hip and resist.

Pain referral pattern: Pain is localized and can be experienced as a full feeling in the rectum. It is also possible that some pain may refer down the back of the ipsilateral thigh.

Needling technique: Ensure the patient is in a secure and comfortable position on the couch, locate the muscle and insert the needle directly into the muscle belly or into a specific point of pain.

Clinical implications: Avoid any deep neurovascular structures such as the sciatic nerve when needling the obturator. If any neurological referral is felt, withdraw the needle and reposition.

Tensor fasciae latae

Palpation: The tensor fasciae latae is a small muscle located on the lateral edge of the anterior hip. The muscle helps to rotate the leg in opposite directions and works in conjunction with the iliotibial band, which is a thick stabilizing tendon. Palpate by side lying, with hip and knee flexed. Stand at the side and face the thigh. Using the palm of the hand, locate the lateral femoral condyle and palpate the fibres along the thigh. Follow the tendon to the belly of the tensor fasciae latae. Resist as the hip abducts.

Pain referral pattern: Pain is localized down the lateral front thigh, towards the knee. It can also extend into the hip and down to the calf muscle.

Needling technique: This technique can be completed with the patient supine or side lying. In either position it is best to support the patient in the normal areas such as the knees. The direction of needling, whether supine or side lying, is to remain perpendicular to the skin.

Clinical implications: None.

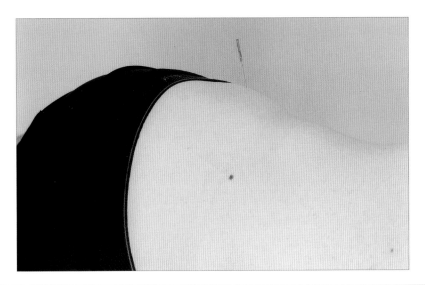

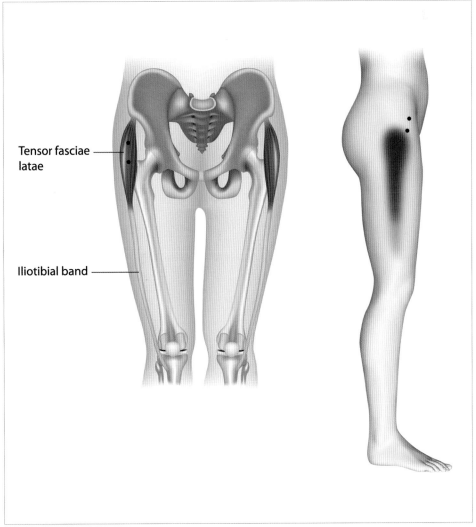

Tensor fasciae latae

Iliotibial band

Figure 11.39 Tensor fasciae latae trigger points

Piriformis

Palpation: Piriformis is a small triangular muscle and one of six hip external rotators located deep in the gluteus maximus and gluteus medius. These rotators help to coordinate stabilization of the hip joint and also position the femoral head. As the most superior external rotator, piriformis is also associated with the sciatic nerve. Palpate by side lying, with hip and knee flexed. Stand at the side and face the thigh to locate the lateral edge of the sacrum.

Following the oblique muscle fibres, slide the fingers towards the greater trochanter, to avoid compressing the sciatic nerve. Palpate and follow the muscle fibres. Resist external rotation of the hip.

Pain referral pattern: Pain is primarily referred to the sacroiliac region and can cause nerve impingement symptoms that include numbness, muscle weakness, tightening and tingling.

Needling technique: The patient may be prone or side lying. Locate the piriformis by using the landmarks of the sacrum and the greater trochanter. Needle the piriformis perpendicular to the table.

Clinical implications: If you irritate the sciatic nerve and the patient's response does not ease, then remove the needle.

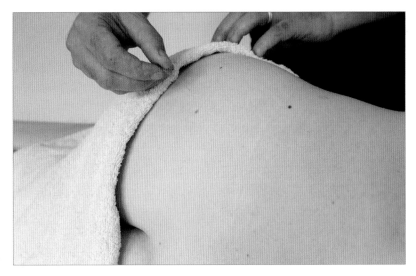

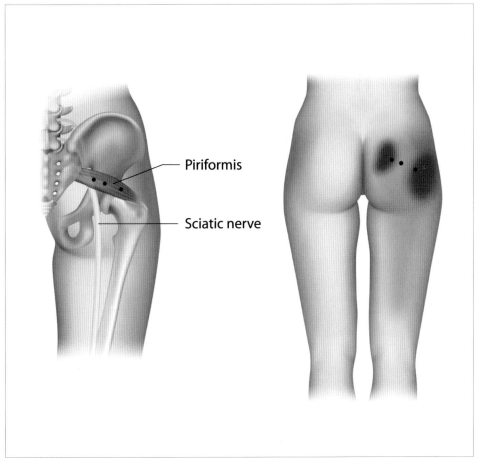

Piriformis

Sciatic nerve

Figure 11.40 Piriformis trigger points

Adductor

Palpation: The adductors are located in the inner hip musculature and originate from the lower pelvic bone to the femur, towards the knee. The group of adductor muscles includes the adductor magnus, which is one of the biggest muscles in the body, the adductor longus, the adductor minimus, the adductor brevis, the gracilis and the pectineus. The muscles work together to facilitate the adduction of the hip joint, and support outward and inward rotation, extension and flexion. Palpate the adductor muscle bellies at the medial side of the thigh. When the knee is extended, the muscles become more stretched and can be palpated.

Pain referral pattern: Pain is localized in the hips and legs, with the adductor longus and adductor brevis referring pain into the groin and down towards the knee and shin.

Needling technique: With the patient supine, position the affected leg in slight hip flexion and external rotation. You may support the patient's leg with yours or with pillows. Insert the needle in an anterior–posterior (AP) direction into the adductor muscle required.

Clinical implications: Avoid needling through the femoral triangle, which is created by the inguinal ligament, sartorius and adductor longus. Many neurovascular structures run through this area and it must be avoided.

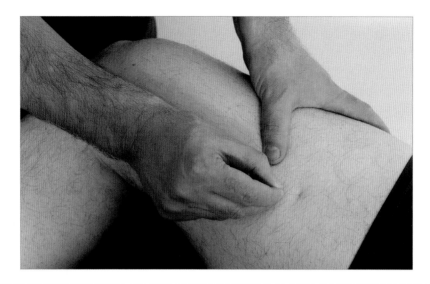

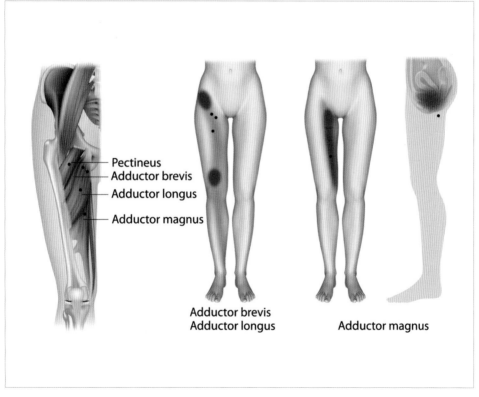

Pectineus
Adductor brevis
Adductor longus
Adductor magnus

Adductor brevis
Adductor longus

Adductor magnus

Figure 11.41 Adductor muscle trigger points

Gracilis

Palpation: The gracilis is a thin strap muscle that extends along the length of the leg, from the point of origin on the pubis to the inside knee joint. Flat palpation, supporting the knee with a pillow, relaxes the distal portion of the adductor longus so that the thin, ropelike gracilis can be palpated from its insertion to the point where it becomes lost in the adductor muscles. The relaxed position offers a moderate stretch.

Pain referral pattern: Pain in the gracilis causes a stinging superficial pain in the medial thigh and down the inside of the leg. The pain can also be constant during rest.

Needling technique: It is best to keep the patient in a supine position to allow you to externally rotate the hip to allow access to the gracilis muscle. Insert the needle perpendicularly into any painful spots within the muscle.

Clinical implications: There are no neurovascular issues within this area, although patients may be prone to bruising on sensitive areas of the body.

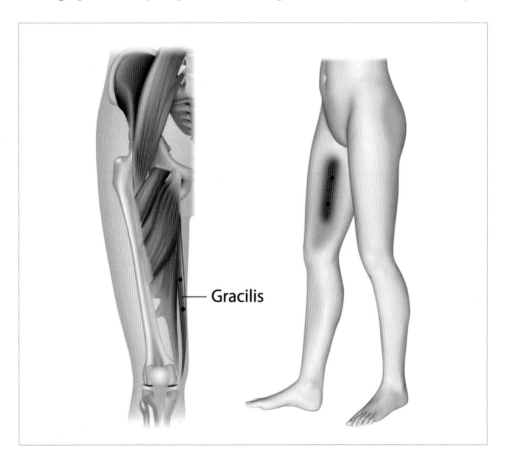

Gracilis

Figure 11.42 Gracilis trigger points

Sartorius

Palpation: The sartorius is a superficial muscle in the interior compartment of the thigh. The longest strap muscle in the body has flattened tendons at the end and reaches down, in a vertical line, from the upper attachment in the anterior superior iliac spine to the gracilis. The muscle facilitates hip and knee flexion, lateral rotation and thigh abduction, which are the movements required for cross-legged sitting. Palpate the sartorius muscle from the origin to its pes anserine tendon insertion point. When lying supine with knee flexed, the muscle can be easily palpated.

Pain referral pattern: The sartorius will primarily refer pain to the leg, ankle and foot. Primary pain is focused in the anterior thigh, with numbness or tingling on the outer thigh. Secondary symptoms include medial thigh pain and anteromedial knee pain.

Needling technique: As with the gracilis, keep the patient in a supine position and needle into the sartorius in a perpendicular angle into the muscle belly.

Clinical implications: Consideration of the femoral nerve, artery and vein should be taken into consideration when needling into this area.

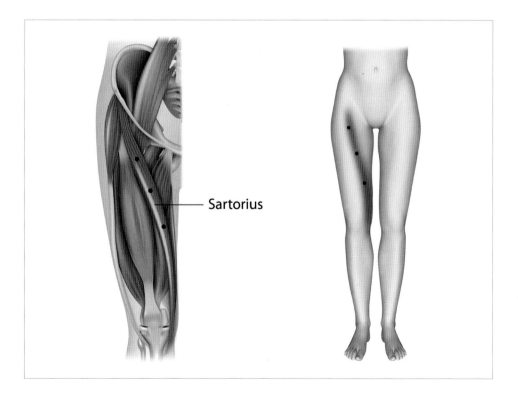

— Sartorius

Figure 11.43 Sartorius trigger points

Semimembranosus, semitendinosus and biceps femoris (hamstrings)

Palpation: The hamstring muscle group consists of three muscles – the semimembranosus, semitendinosus and biceps femoris. The semimembranosus muscle has a broad belly and is located on the medial aspect of the posterior thigh. It runs from the ischial tuberosity of the pelvis.

The semitendinosus muscle also originates from the ischial tuberosity of the pelvis and is located on the same aspect. Contraction of the hamstrings causes extension of the thigh, at the hip. Once the hip is extended, these muscles help with medial rotation and rotate the leg at the knee when the knee is flexed. To palpate in prone position, stand at the side of the table and use one hand to add resistance. Locate the large distal tendon in the posterior knee and the shared origin. Palpate the fibres of the muscles.

The biceps femoris is located in the back of the thigh. The lateral muscle is superficial in the posterolateral thigh and has two heads. The long head posteriorly crosses the hip joint and flexes the leg at the knee joint. The short head cannot extend the thigh and originates distal to the femoral attachment of the gluteus maximus. The biceps femoris is the only muscle that can laterally rotate the legs and medially rotate the thigh. In prone position, partially flex at the knee and palpate the muscle from the point of origin to insertion on the lateral side. Resist knee flexion and palpate the muscle toward the head of the fibula.

Pain referral pattern: The hamstring group of muscles is the most overworked in the human body and has a referred pain pattern that concentrates on two areas. Medial pain refers pain upwards into the upper posterior thigh region and down the back of the thigh to the medial calf area. Lateral pain primarily refers to the back of the knee, with secondary referral to the back of the thigh and lower back.

Needling technique: The patient should be in a comfortable prone position. Place a pillow under the patient's legs if needed. Locate the muscle directly, and on palpation identify painful spots within the muscle belly. A needle can be inserted in the biceps femoris in a perpendicular angle.

Clinical implications: There is a theoretical risk of hitting the sciatic nerve in the posterior aspect of the leg, although this thick nerve lies deep to the muscle. To avoid the sciatic nerve, focus on needling the muscle superficially at an oblique angle.

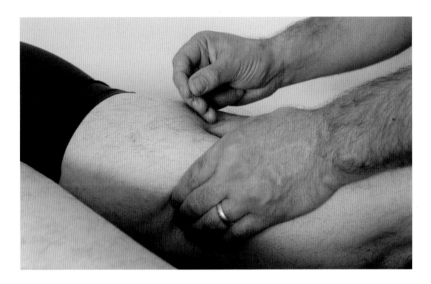

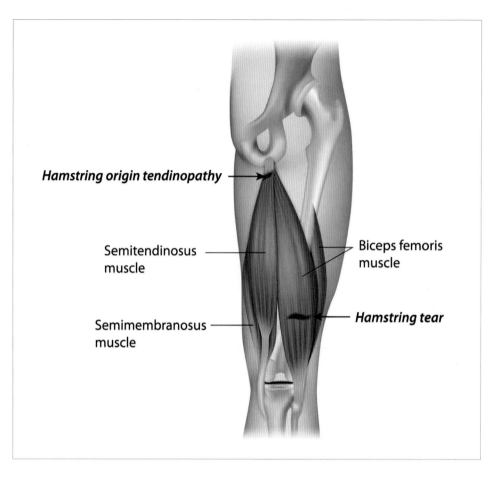

Figure 11.44 Hamstring injury (right leg, dorsal view)

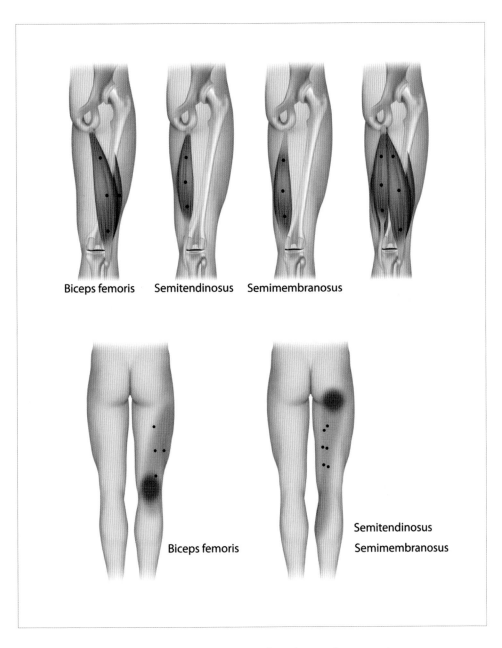

Biceps femoris   Semitendinosus   Semimembranosus

Biceps femoris

Semitendinosus
Semimembranosus

Figure 11.45 Hamstring trigger points

Popliteus

Palpation: The popliteus muscle originates from three points – the lateral femoral condyle, fibula and posterior horn of the lateral meniscus. The muscle rises from the proximal tibia and inserts into the posterior surface of the tibia, above the soleus. The thin and flat triangular popliteus muscle wraps around the lower section of the femur and provides flexion of the knee joint and lateral rotation of the femur. The muscle is most accessible at the lower medial end and upper lateral end of the muscle belly. In prone position, palpate directly between the semitendinosus tendon and medial head of the gastrocnemius muscle. Flex the knee, and the foot at the ankle, to slacken the muscles. The soleus muscle can be laterally displaced to partially uncover the popliteus.

Pain referral pattern: Popliteus primary pain referral is localized in the leg, ankle and foot and refers to posterior knee pain.

Needling technique: With the patient either prone or side lying, locate the muscle behind the posterior aspect of the knee. Use an inferior needling technique to needle the muscle laterally, avoiding deep perpendicular needling of the posterior knee.

Clinical implications: Be aware of the neurovascular bundle which sits just behind the popliteus muscle. Using an inferior technique to needle the muscle laterally will avoid contacting this delicate structure. If the patient does feel a strong referral from the nerve, then remove and replace the needle.

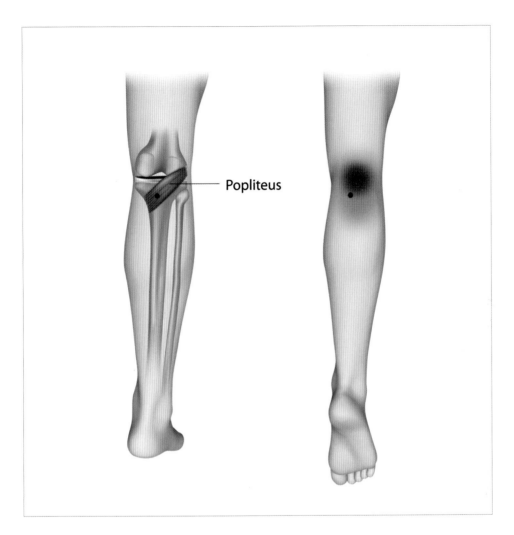

Figure 11.46 Popliteus trigger point

Gastrocnemius and soleus

Palpation: The gastrocnemius and soleus muscles are located in the calf region and are known as the tricep surae muscles. The muscles work together as plantar flexors, which bend the foot back at the ankle joint. This also causes the leg to flex at the knee and results in propulsion and stabilization. The gastrocnemius is the largest calf muscle and is positioned over the soleus muscle.

It originates from the knee and runs to the ankle joint. The gastrocnemius has two parallel muscle bellies that merge together mid-calf. The soleus has multiple origin points, with fibres merging into a large tendon and inserting into the heel bone. Palpate the entire length of the calf. Extend the knee in prone position and resist. Palpate the medial and lateral heads and the attachment on the heel.

Pain referral pattern: The gastrocnemius and soleus muscles have an extended pain referral pattern for the whole of the calf region, including the outside calf. Pain concentrates in the instep of the foot and can also extend upwards to the back of the thigh. Secondary pain is referred to the back of the knee.

Needling technique: With the patient prone or side lying, palpate the gastrocnemius muscle and locate specific points of pain, needling in a perpendicular angle into the centre bulk of the muscle. With the soleus, palpate and locate the target area, and insert the needle in either the lateral or medial side of the calf and needle towards the soleus.

Clinical implications: There are several nerves which run through the lower extremity, and these should be avoided. If the patient feels an electrical referral, then the needles should be removed and replaced slightly away from the painful spot.

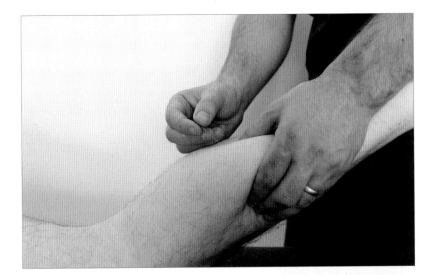

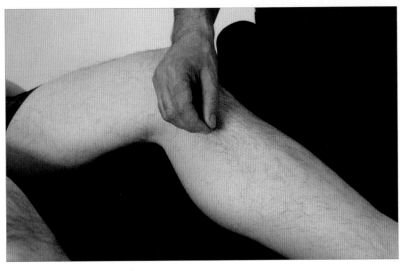

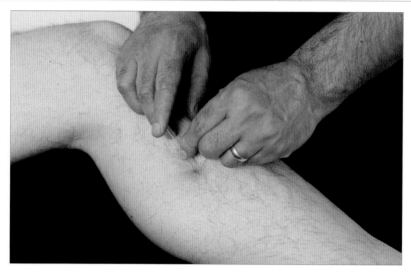

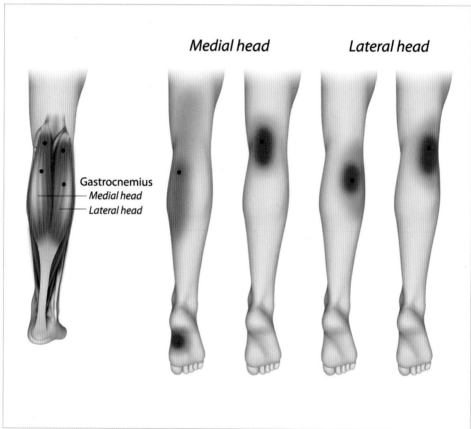

Figure 11.47 Gastrocnemius trigger points

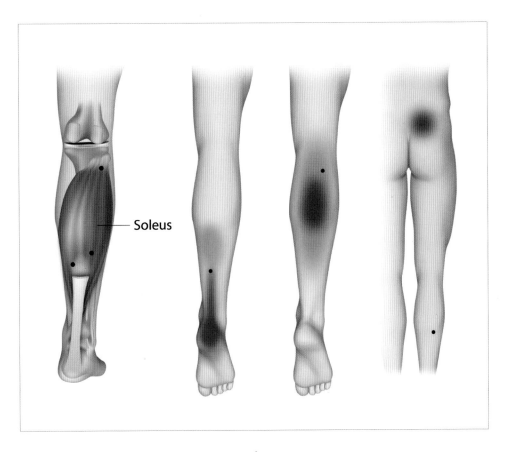

Figure 11.48 Soleus trigger points

Plantaris

Palpation: The small plantaris muscle is located in the posterior aspect of the leg, and forms part of the posterosuperficial compartment of the calf. Along with the gastrocnemius and soleus, the thin muscle belly and long thin tendon make up the triceps surae muscle.

The plantaris originates from the lateral supracondylar line of the femur and from the oblique popliteal ligament located in the posterior aspect of the knee. Palpation of the muscle is possible in the popliteal fossa and the medial aspect of the common tendon. In prone position, flex the leg and cover the heel with the distal hand. Use the forearm to create resistance for the foot and knee flexion. Palpate the muscle in the popliteal fossa and Achilles tendon.

Pain referral pattern: The plantaris primarily refers pain in the posterior aspect and plantar surface of the heel. This can include the distal end of the Achilles tendon and the sacroiliac joints on the same side of the body. Pain is referred to the posterior of the knee and into the calf region.

Needling technique: Locate the upper lateral head of the gastrocnemius muscle and locate the plantaris muscle. Needle into the muscle in either a perpendicular or lateral direction.

Clinical implications: Be cautious around the tibial and peroneal nerves. If the patient feels a strong referral, then the needle should be removed and replaced nearby.

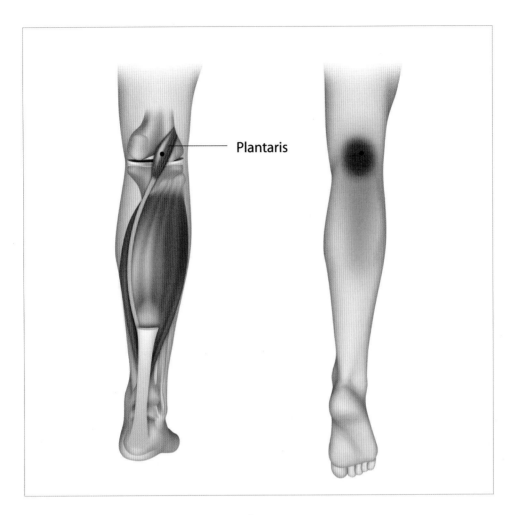

Plantaris

Figure 11.49 Plantaris trigger point

Peroneals

Palpation: The peroneal muscle group is made up of two muscles – the peroneus longus and peroneus brevis – and is located within the peroneal compartment, in the lower leg region. The muscles can be easily seen when the foot is lowered, as they form the surface of the lateral lower leg. The muscle tendons run towards the foot behind the lateral malleolus and ventrally along the edge of the foot. The peroneus longus and peroneus brevis are responsible for moving the upper and lower ankle joints. Palpate the hollow behind the malleolus and the tendons that pass under and over the peroneal tubercle. The peroneals brevis can be palpated to its insertion.

Pain referral pattern: The primary peroneal pain refers over the lateral malleolus of the ankle and over the lateral aspect of the foot and lateral heel region. The outside edge of the shin is a secondary referral site.

Needling technique: Locate the muscle belly and angle the needle towards the fibula, with the needle being inserted in a perpendicular angle towards the skin.

Clinical implications: A caution is the location of the common peroneal nerve which sits underneath the muscle. The more superficial peroneus nerve also lies within the area. Avoid direct contact of the nerve; and if the patient indicates a strong electrical referral, then the needle should be removed and replaced nearby.

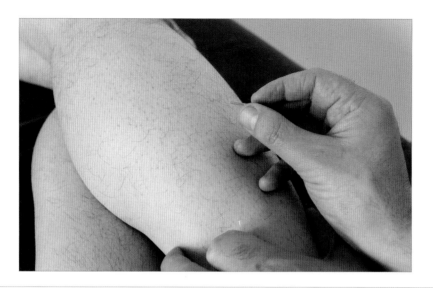

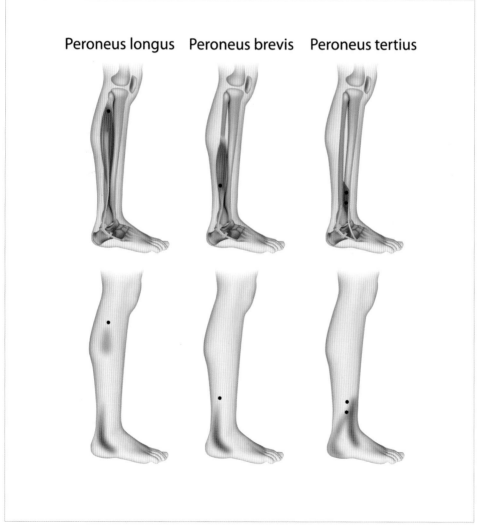

Peroneus longus   Peroneus brevis   Peroneus tertius

Figure 11.50 Peroneal muscle trigger points

Tibialis anterior and posterior

Palpation: The tibialis anterior is located in the front of the leg. The large superficial muscle originates close to the lateral tibial condyle and inserts on the foot. Together with the peroneus longus, which inserts at the base of the foot, the tibialis anterior forms a stirrup that loops around the midfoot. The muscles control movement of the foot.

The tibialis anterior adjusts its function according to the position of the foot and also supports the medial arch. To palpate, stand at the feet and use the thumb to locate the lateral edge of the tibial shaft. Laterally slide onto the muscle belly and continue to palpate towards the front of the ankle and arch. Resist for ankle dorsiflexion and inversion.

Pain referral pattern: As a great deal of stress is put on the front of the tibialis anterior, pain is referred to the shin, ankle or foot. The pain starts gradually and can worsen over time due to aggravated activity. The tibialis anterior tendon is a secondary referral site.

Needling technique: With the patient supine or side lying, locate the bulk of the tibialis anterior or needle directly into any tender spots identified in a perpendicular manner. Angle the needle slightly medially to avoid the underlying neurovascular bundle.

Clinical implications: Deep to the tibialis anterior lies the peroneal nerve and the tibial artery and vein. Needling at a medial angle will limit or avoid this structure.

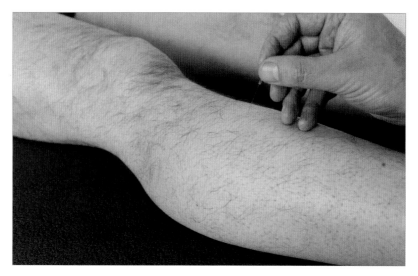

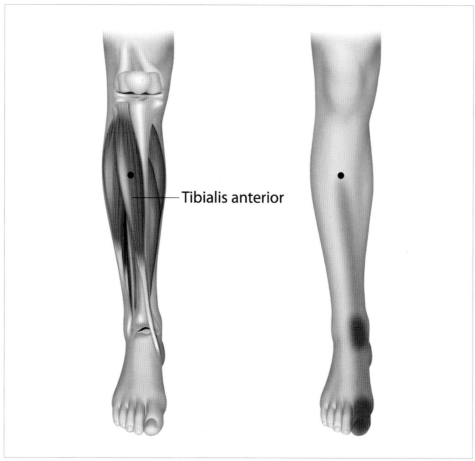

Tibialis anterior

Figure 11.51 Tibialis anterior trigger point

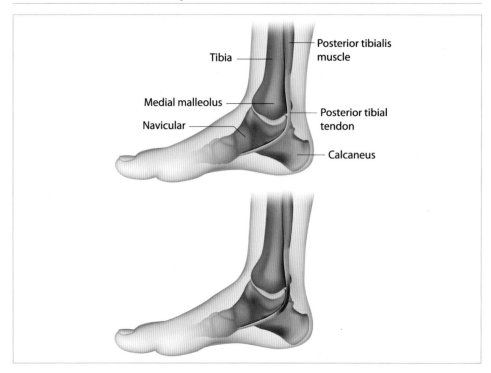

Figure 11.52 Posterior tibial tendon dysfunction

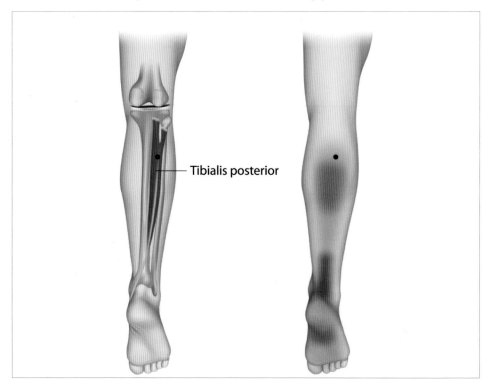

Figure 11.53 Tibialis posterior trigger point

Chapter 12

Electroacupuncture

Introduction

The use of electrotherapy within medicine is not a new concept; indeed, it has a long history of genuine medical application. The earliest reference of its application was found in ancient Greece, where electric eels were used in clinical footbaths to relieve pain and enhance blood circulation (Garrison 1921). Today, electrotherapy is applied with a scientific basis and has a number of therapeutic uses, including wound healing, pain control and fracture repair (Gildenberg 2006).

Electroacupuncture (EA) is a technique of acupuncture which utilizes the electrical stimulation of needles. This chapter reviews the theoretical mechanisms of EA, the scientific evidence behind its effectiveness, its clinical implications, safety guidelines and some practical suggestions for use in clinic.

What is electroacupuncture?

EA is a modified form of traditional manual acupuncture in which an electrical current is applied between pairs of acupuncture needles using a device which controls the frequency and strength of the electrical current being delivered. During a standard EA session, several needle pairs can be stimulated simultaneously, usually for 10–20 minutes, but rarely exceeding 30 minutes (Noordergraaf and Silage 1973).

The use of electrotherapy has a long history, but today's practice owes much to the experimentation in China post-1950 (Dharmananda 2002). Professor Ji-Sheng Han from Beijing Medical University conducted a series of experiments to produce analgesia. This discovery led to EA devices being used on patients undergoing surgery, to the extent that 11 per cent of patients did not require any anaesthetic. This was widely misreported, with news spreading that in China patients were undergoing surgery without anaesthesia. Often EA was supplemented with opiates and anaesthetics, giving the impression that patients were awake with no anaesthesia. It was these reports and the rise in acupuncture use in general during the Cultural Revolution that renewed the interest in EA in the West. Typically EA is no longer used as an analgesic substitute but is still used in the reduction of pain pre- and post-surgery.

Today EA is mainly used as an effective alternative and complementary treatment to treat acute and chronic pain. It is reported to produce analgesia in chronic pain conditions where manual acupuncture (MA) has been shown to be ineffective. Lin and Chen (2008) suggest that the electrical stimulation of acupuncture points provides the therapeutic effects of MA and transcutaneous electric nerve stimulation (TENS) combined. In contrast to classical acupuncture, EA is preferred by most studies, since it can be easily standardized by characteristics such as frequency, waveform and voltage.

EA uses the same acupuncture points as MA to attain deqi, a sensation of heaviness, soreness or numbness (Ahn *et al.* 2008); however, Dharmananda (2002) states that there are some benefits of using EA over MA:

- It substitutes the need for the prolonged manual manipulation of needles by providing a continued stimulus.

- It affords the exact amount of needle stimulation required to a patient.

- It can generate a much stronger stimulation, if needed, without eliciting any tissue damage which may be associated with the manual manoeuvring of needles.

- It provides more flexibility in controlling the stimulus frequency and amount than MA.

EA may have greater effects than MA in many situations, including increased and sustained pain reduction, increased tissue repair and a greater effect on the immune system. There is debate as to whether or not it is important to obtain a local twitch response before applying EA. The argument for obtaining deqi is that this would enhance the therapeutic effect, activating the potential effects of both MA and EA. For many patients, acupuncture may be a last resort, particularly for those being classified as chronic pain patients, so obtaining acupuncture's effects via electrical stimulation is necessary if clinical changes are sought quickly and efficiently.

The use of EA can be thought of as a modern scientific extension of acupuncture. As Woolf (1984, p.679) states: 'The ability for a clinician to reduce pain in a patient by exploiting the patient's own built-in neurophysiologic mechanisms must rank as one of modern science's greatest achievements.'

EA also has similarities with TENS. A TENS machine is similar to an EA machine in that it is a small, battery-operated device that has leads connected to electrodes. The electrodes are connected to adhesive pads which are placed on the skin, delivering the electric current. TENS is probably the more frequently used electrotherapy due to it being non-invasive and easy to administer. EA on the other hand is an invasive procedure which delivers the current through the skin rather than across it. Mayor (2007) claims that this has advantages over TENS as EA will need less current to achieve motor stimulation, the waveform is less distorted and deeper muscle afferents can be stimulated without pain from cutaneous C-fibres (a cutaneous receptor is a type of sensory receptor found in the dermis or epidermis). EA, however, will cause a degree of local tissue inflammation due to its invasive nature, whereas TENS would not.

Common medical conditions that EA has been used to treat include the following.

Relief of acute pain

- Musculoskeletal pain
- Tendinopathies
- Post-operative pain
- Labour pain
- Dysmenorrhoea
- Bone fractures
- Dental pain

Relief of chronic pain

- Low back pain

- Arthritis

- Phantom pain

- Post-operative pain

- Trigeminal neuralgia

- Peripheral nerve injuries

- Facial pain

- Neurological conditions, for example Parkinson's and stroke

Other effects of EA

- Modulation of immune, endocrine and circulatory systems

- Antiemetic effects, including nausea associated with chemotherapy and morning sickness

Other improvements useful in MSK conditions

- Acceleration of tissue repair by increasing circulation

- Increase in blood flow

- Increased muscle strengthening

- Improved muscle control

- Reduction of muscle spasticity

- Treatment of denervated muscle – compression injuries only

- Improved healing of wounds, ulcers and scar tissue

Physiological mechanisms of electroacupuncture

Over the past decades, many studies have suggested various mechanisms of EA; however, so far no satisfactory consensus has been reached. Moreover, EA has a wide variety of clinical applications, which in turn make it even more difficult to elucidate the exact mechanism of action. Nevertheless, a number of researchers have progressively investigated the physiological mechanisms behind its various applications. To date, pain management is one of its most thoroughly studied applications (Lee, LaRiccia and Newberg 2004a, b).

Mechanism of EA in pain control

EA induces its analgesic effects via neuronal mechanisms associated with both the peripheral nervous system (PNS) and central nervous system (CNS), involving many brain regions as well as different neurotransmitters and modulators (Hsieh *et al.* 2000; Lianfang 1987; Pomeranz, Cheng and Law 1977). Studies have hypothesized that a number of signalling molecules, such as endogenous opioid peptides, cholecystokinin octapeptide, noradrenalin, serotonin, dopamine, glutamate, γ-amino-butyric acid and other bioactive substances, may have direct influence in these mechanisms (Leung 2012; Yoo *et al.* 2011; Zhao 2008). In addition, Lin and Chen (2008) postulated that several pain pathways might be involved, including the hypothalamus–pituitary–adrenal (HPA) axis, the autonomic nervous system (ANS) and the descending inhibitory pathway (hypothalamus–periaqueductal grey area–raphe nucleus–spinal cord).

However, scientific evidence for EA's influence on HPA and ANS is still limited; therefore, this section will particularly concentrate on the neural mechanisms of EA that have been strongly proposed as possible explanations for its analgesic effects.

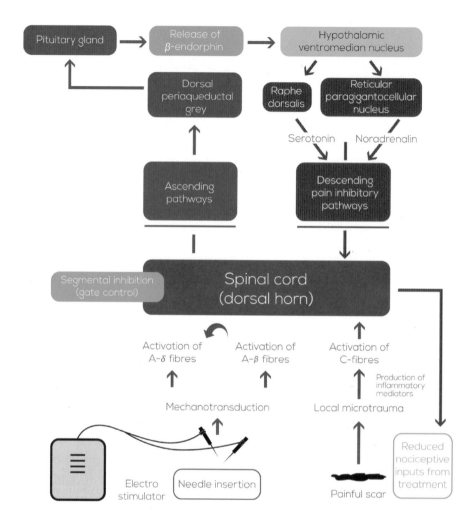

Figure 12.1 Schematic diagram of the physiological mechanisms of EA-induced analgesia (derived from Cagnie et al. 2013; Leung 2012; Okada and Kawakita 2009)
Blue arrows = activation; red arrows = inhibition

Gate control theory

The segmental mechanism of EA is frequently explained by Melzack and Wall's (1967) gate control theory, which proposes that A-δ and C sensory fibres open the substantia gelatinosa (SG) layer located in the dorsal horn of the spinal cord, while A-β fibres or descending inhibition block the layer. Based on this theory, it has long been postulated that low-frequency electrical stimulation of needles excites A-β fibres and this in turn blocks A-δ and C-fibres in the same segment of the spinal cord that transmit nociceptive signals to the brain (Pyne and Shenker 2008). In support of this hypothesis, evidence has already demonstrated that EA-induced stimulation of A-β fibres is capable of producing analgesia (Pomeranz and Paley 1979; Chung *et al.* 1984; Toda 2002); however, it is also reported that excitation of some A-δ fibres in addition to A-β fibres produces a more potent analgesia (Leung *et al.* 2005).

Endorphins theory

The release of various endorphins has been one of the leading theories regarding EA-induced analgesia. The theory hypothesizes that the analgesic effects of EA result from the release of endogenous opiates and their receptors. Pomeranz and Chiu (1976) first proposed this hypothesis based on their finding in mice that naloxone, an antagonist to opiate (morphine-like substrate), is able to block or reverse the analgesic effect of acupuncture. Later, Mayer, Price and Rafii (1977) reported a similar result of naloxone administration in humans; consequently, the release of morphine-like substrate in the CNS was presumed to be a possible mechanism of EA. Since the proposal of this theory, evidence from a number of both human and animal studies has further clarified the role of endogenous opiates.

Furthermore, it is suggested that electrical stimulation of needles at different frequencies can vary the type of endogenous endorphine released (Chen and Han 1992). Guo *et al.* (1996) showed that low-frequency EA (2 Hz) enhances the expression of enkephalin precursor proteins, while high-frequency EA (100 Hz) increases the expression of dynorphin precursors. Later, Han *et al.* (1999) and Huang *et al.* (2004), based on their results in human volunteers, concluded that low-frequency EA mediates μ- and δ-opioid receptors and stimulates the release of β-endorphin, enkephalin and endomorphin. In addition, Han (2003) confirmed that high-frequency EA mediates the κ-opioid receptor and releases dynorphin.

Serotonin theory

Serotonin and its receptors in the CNS have been presumed to play an important role in EA-induced analgesia, collaborating with endogenous opiates. The theory of a serotonergic descending inhibitory pathway of EA was developed when Tsai, Chen and Lin (1989) found that p-chlorophenylalanine, a serotonin synthesis inhibitor, diminished the analgesic effect of acupuncture analgesia.

After this finding, much research was done to elucidate the serotonergic mechanism of EA. Takagi and Yonehara (1998), based on their study on the tooth pulp of rabbits, reported that antagonists of the serotonin receptor subtype are associated with an EA-induced block of acute nociceptive impulses. Baek, Yang and Park (2005) found that pargyline, a monoamine oxidase inhibitor, facilitates serotonin receptor degradation, which in turn potentiates the analgesic effect of EA.

Noradrenalin theory

Noradrenalin has been seen to act differently at the spinal and supraspinal levels. Yoo *et al.* (2011) found that administration of noradrenalin precursor blocks EA-induced analgesia, whereas intrathecal injection potentiates it. In addition, several lines of evidence reported that, in the spinal dorsal horn, 1-adrenergic receptors facilitate nociceptive signalling, while 2-adrenergic receptors suppress it. For example, in rats with neuropathic pain, Kim *et al.* (2005) found that antagonists of 2-adrenergic receptors inhibited the analgesic effects of EA on cold allodynia.

Habituation and sensitization

Chronic pain patients display features of central hypersensitivity with changes in the CNS after peripheral injury. Prolonged afferent nociceptive input may induce a reversible increase in the excitability of central sensory neurons with an expansion of the receptive field, resulting in changing the sensory response elicited by normal inputs (Curatolo, Arendt-Nielsen and Petersen-Felix 2006).

Habituation occurs when an organism decreases or ceases to respond to a stimulus after repeated presentations. Habituation can be thought of as the opposite of sensitization: the habituation process is decremental; whereas the sensitization process is incremental, enhancing the tendency to respond. The discovery of neuroplasticity that the CNS is able to change neural pathways and synapses due to changes may be advantageous when using EA. EA provides regular signals, and sustained stimulation to an area leads to habituation. The possibility exists therefore that EA leads to habituation, reversing sensitization. However, there is not much evidence to support the presumption that acupuncture analgesia is due to the habituation effects of acupuncture stimulation, so therefore more research is needed in this area.

The parameters of electroacupuncture

EA involves electrophysical, electrochemical and electrothermal phenomena (Cameron 2012); its therapeutic effects depend on a number of factors, including the type of waveform, intensity, frequency, duration and course of electric flow to the particular tissue type in which it is applied (Silvério-Lopes 2011). These factors can alter the desired clinical effects during a typical session if EA is not administered correctly to the patient.

Frequency

Frequency, from the physics perspective, refers to the number of cycles delivered per second. It is measured in units of Hertz (Hz). Mathematically, each single cycle is measured as a unit of time (microsecond), so if a pulsation has a cycle of 0.25 seconds (i.e. occurring four times per second), it is expressed as 4 Hz (Walsh and Berry 2010).

Figure 12.2 shows a visual representation of an electric current. The vertical axis is the amplitude (the strength of the current), which is adjusted by the intensity controls on the EA machine. Time is on the horizontal axis. The wave in this example begins above the baseline and is the strength of the wave moving in one direction, and below the baseline as it moves in the other direction. One complete cycle is measured as 1 Hz. In EA, a low frequency would be around 2–10 Hz and a high frequency would be 50–200 Hz (Mayor 2007a).

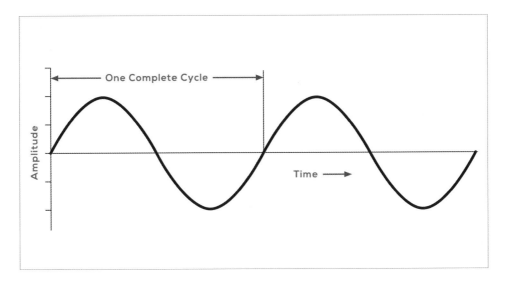

Figure 12.2 An electric current

Scientific research has shown that there is a strong relationship between frequency and release of endogenous opioids, which play a major role in EA-induced analgesia. Frequency-dependent EA studies conducted on rats have reported the release of a number of biochemical substances at different frequencies, such as enkephalin, β-endorphin and endomorphin at 2 Hz (Han 2004); dynorphin at 100 Hz (Han 2003); enkephalin and dynorphin at 2 and 100 Hz (Zhang *et al.* 2005b); and substance P (SP) at 10 Hz (Zhang *et al.* 2005a).

Table 12.1 EA-induced release of biochemical substances at different frequencies

Frequencies (Hz)	Enkephalin	ß-endorphin	Endomorphin	Dynorphin	SP	Cholecystokinin octapeptide
2	+	+	+			
4			+	+		
10					+	
15	+	+		+		
100			+	+		+

Adapted from Han 2004; Huang et al. 2004 and Silvério-Lopes 2011.

Different frequencies and intensities will produce different physiological responses, and it is important to monitor the patient during an EA treatment and elicit these both verbally and by observation of the patient's response. Low frequency will often produce muscle twitching and contraction (from the activation of motor neurons). Higher frequencies will often produce numbness and tingling due to sensory nerve activation and can be a very pleasant and relaxing sensation, if not slightly unusual. Warmth can signal increased circulation in an area (Walsh and Berry 2010). From selecting different frequencies, observing the physical response and monitoring the patient, it is likely that the correct dose is being administered, resulting in the desired outcome.

Lee (2012) offers some sound practical advice on the use of frequency by using different combinations of high and low frequencies at different stages of treatment. He starts with a high frequency to reduce overall pain, with a setting of 100/33 Hz. Once pain has reduced, he then uses a low frequency of 10/3 Hz to restore normal muscle functioning.

For an in-depth resource on the use of EA for certain conditions, the reader is encouraged to consult the companion website to Mayor (2007b). This database presents clinical studies that have been carried out on EA and other non-traditional acupuncture-based interventions in a succinct and accessible form.

Waveforms used in EA

Most of the modern EA machines allow the therapist to monitor the intensity and frequency only, though some devices also allow adjusting the wave formation, which can have different therapeutic effects. These machines often have a fixed output pulse width (between 0.2ms and 0.4ms) and waveforms. In EA, however, biphasic square waves are mostly used, although some machines generate spike or other waveforms (Mayor 2007a). Some examples of waveforms are shown in Figure 12.3.

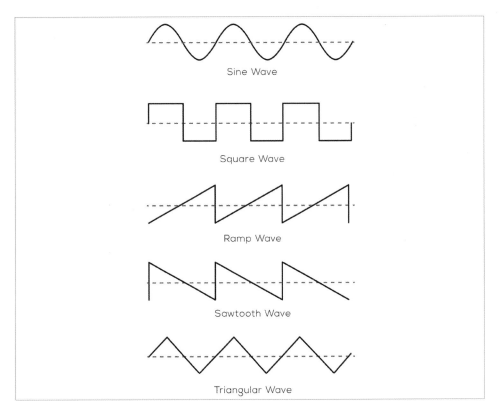

Sine Wave

Square Wave

Ramp Wave

Sawtooth Wave

Triangular Wave

Figure 12.3 Examples of waveforms

Stimulation may be continuous, intermittent (burst), dense–disperse or otherwise modulated (see Figure 12.4).

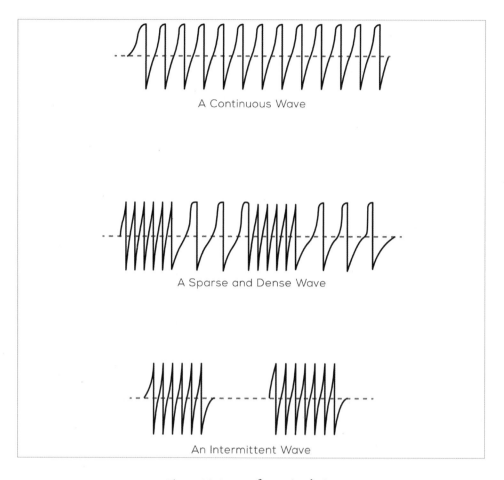

Figure 12.4 Waveform stimulation

A continuous wave is a uniform wave with a constant amplitude and frequency that therefore does not change over time. It is very similar to what Chinese acupuncturists try to administer by MA. The advantage of using this waveform in EA is that it is well tolerated by patients and the stimulus is quickly adapted. However, high intensity may be required to maximize its therapeutic effects (Mayor 2007b).

An intermittent, or discontinuous, wave flows at irregular intervals and appears on and off rhythmically. It provides a series of equally spaced pulses but with gaps of inactivity. Patients also usually adapt to this stimulus (Paraskevaidis *et al.* 1999).

A dense–disperse wave is a combination of two waves (disperse and dense) which appear alternately, lasting about 1.5s, to prevent the body's adaptation to the stimulation. Dense–disperse waves provide equally proportioned periods of high- and low-frequency pulsations. They work at both sensory and motor neuronal levels and stimulate endogenous pain suppressants (Yang *et al.* 2007).

Table 12.2 Characteristics of dense and disperse waves

Waveform type	Dense wave (continuous)	Disperse wave (continuous)
Frequency	High frequency: 50–100 pulses per second	Low frequency: 2–5 pulses per second
Function	• Inhibits sensory nerves and motor nerves • Relieves spasm of the muscles and blood vessels	• Induces the contraction of muscles • Enhances the tension of muscles and ligaments
Indication	Pain relief, trauma	Paralysis, injury of muscle, ligament and joints

Intensity

In EA, the term 'intensity' usually refers to a measure of current or voltage. The intensity of the electrical current in acupoints has a distinct effect on the patient's physiological responses, and can be seen in subtle changes (Walsh and Berry 2010). In addition, the strength of sensation experienced by the patient relies on intensity more than on frequency.

The majority of devices on the market use an alternating current (AC), since it ensures more safety for the patient than a direct current (DC). In EA, an AC prevents the build-up of any electron charge at the points of contact, while a DC can produce excessive heat, which may cause more pain and discomfort. In general, the order of 12mA (milliamperes) or 9V (volts) may be the maximum intensity, but these figures may vary significantly depending on equipment design (Mayor 2007a).

But not too intense...

The intensity of stimulus should be the minimum required for the patient to experience its effect. If the minimum amount results in a painful reaction, the practitioner should provide adequate care to restrict the muscle twitching to a mild response. The face and areas below the elbow and knee are highly sensitive to electrical stimulation; therefore, these areas should be stimulated at a very low intensity. In addition, patients who are taking EA for the first time should receive MA first, so that suitability and tolerance for EA can be ensured (Dharmananda 2002).

No pain, no gain...?

At no time should there be pain during EA.

The intensity controls should only be increased in minute adjustments, and the patient's response should be monitored with every adjustment. There can be a very small increase in intensity which will result in a sudden, often painful, response in the patient. EA machines do not have a linear relationship between their intensity settings and the amplitude of stimulation; that is, each degree of movement on the intensity dial is not equivalent to a similar increase in pulse amplitude.

Walsh and Berry (2010) draw attention to the fact that devices can change their electrical output depending on battery power, with quicker responses occurring with charged batteries with a relatively low intensity setting, while the same batteries that are low in power will require a higher intensity setting before achieving the same result.

Longer distances between needles may require a higher intensity when increased absorption will occur, as energy needs to overcome internal friction that exists in tissue while travelling through it. However, again closely monitor your patient's response when increasing the intensity.

Safety of electroacupuncture

EA is safe when conducted by a trained practitioner, with relatively low incidence of side effects (MacPherson *et al.* 2004). Although some blood-borne diseases such as hepatitis and HIV have been reported, these are rare, as disposable acupuncture needles are now widely used. Other adverse reactions reported include broken needles, bleeding, infection, nerve damage, cardiac tamponade, contact dermatitis and punctures of organs (Lee *et al.* 2004b).

Researchers have stated that side effects of EA usually occur as a result of bad practice by a practitioner who has not been properly trained. However, some mild, temporary reactions may occur in some cases despite proper administration of EA by a qualified practitioner. These include pain at the point of a needle's puncture, bleeding or bruising from the puncture point, drowsiness, feeling unwell, dizziness or fainting, and worsening of pre-existing symptoms (Cummings 2011).

Table 12.3 Side effects of EA

Majority of cases	Commonly (about 1–10%)	Rarely (less than 1%)
None	• Bleeding • Haematoma • Pain at needling site	• Hepatitis or HIV transmission • Needle stick injury • Nerve damage and paraesthesias • Pneumothoraces • Cardiac tamponade • Punctures of organs • Infection • Contact dermatitis • Nausea and vomiting

Adapted from Lee et al. 2004b.

Contraindications

According to the World Health Organization (1999), EA should be avoided in the following conditions:

- pacemaker in situ

- uterus or pelvic girdle in pregnancy

- pregnancy (first trimester)

- impaired circulation

- severe arterial disease

- bleeding disorders

- spontaneous bleeding or bruising

- undiagnosed fever

- unstable diabetes

- severe skin lesions

- malignant tumours

- unstable epilepsy or history of unexplained convulsions

- medical emergencies and surgical conditions

- needle phobia or overanxiousness.

In addition, needling should be avoided in certain areas of the body. These include:

- fontanelle in babies

- external genitalia

- anterior portion of the neck

- broken, fragile, inflamed or infected skin

- areas affected by lymphedema

- nipples

- uterine innervations segment (in pregnant women)

- umbilicus

- eyeball.

Precautions

- Acupuncture needles should not be moved abruptly, since this may result in displaced or lost needles.

- Galvanic current should be used for only a very short period of time.

- Electrical current should not be passed through, near or around a fracture.

- Appropriate care should be taken if the patient has a compromised lymphatic system or is immunosuppressed through illness or medication.

- Electrical stimulation of needles should be carefully monitored to prevent neural injury.

- Appropriate care should be taken if sensory nerve damage is present.

- Special care should be taken in areas that have poor circulation because these areas often heal poorly and have collateral blood vessels that may bleed.

- Careful monitoring must be carried out if the patient has a form of cardiac arrhythmia, so that this is not aggravated.

- EA practitioners should be wary of metal piercings and must not pass current through metal implants and joints.

- Low-frequency stimulation may change original needle position. Cases have been reported where needles have been further drawn into the body, or forced out, due to muscle contraction.

Consent and practicalities for EA treatment

- The EA practitioner should inform the patient about all treatment options. The patient should be given clear details of the offered treatment and what it involves.

- The patient's written informed consent must be documented prior to treatment. Children (below 16 years of age) should not be treated unless written consent is taken from a parent or guardian.

- The patient must participate in a primary health check-up or complete a checklist to identify possible contraindications or cautions to treatment.

- The EA practitioner should advise the patient to assume a comfortable posture before needling. The patient should be requested to remain relaxed and not to change position abruptly during treatment.

- The EA practitioner should inform the patient about the possibility of transient symptoms during and after treatment, including faintness, fatigue, bruising or the temporary aggravation of symptoms.

- The practitioner should inform the patient that, during the needling, he/she may experience local or distal 'tingling' or 'sporadic' muscle contractions, and that this is a normal reaction of needling.

- The intensity of the stimulation should be carefully monitored. The stimulation intensity should never reach the level of pain. If it becomes uncomfortable or painful for the patient, it should be either reduced or stopped, depending on the severity.

- Once the treatment is finished, post-treatment care is recommended. The patient should be informed that he/she might feel light-headed, stiff and sore for 24–48 hours.

- Adequate records of all procedures must be kept in a safe and secure manner.

Beginning EA treatment

- Needle acupuncture points as chosen.

- Attach clips to needles.

- Choose frequency and pulse duration on the EA machine.

- Ensure the machine is at zero before switching on.

- Tell the patient that you are about to begin treatment and that they should inform you of any sensations felt; it should not be painful.

- Slowly turn on intensity and monitor the patient for verbal and non-verbal signs; monitor throughout treatment and change intensity settings if too strong.

At the end of treatment

- Slowly turn down intensity controls to zero.

- Switch off the EA machine.

- Disconnect all leads, taking care not to stimulate/knock needles.

- Remove needles as standard practice and dispose of accordingly.

- Check that all needles have been removed.

- Inform the patient that all needles have been removed.

- Let the patient rest for a few minutes and monitor them as they get up from the couch.

- Clean crocodile clips if necessary and pack away leads for next time.

- Inform the patient of any effects of treatment.

Basic EA machine guidelines

Irrespective of the EA/TENS device used, there are a number of important variables that practitioners should be aware of when setting up their machine for treatment. These settings include the intensity, frequency and mode of delivery. Basic EA machines are relatively cheap: a good example is the AWQ-104E Chinese machine, which is small enough to be portable, has four outputs and has a digital display to depict the frequency of stimulation during operation. More expensive machines will have more outputs and greater control over the waveforms used. Generally speaking, though, EA machines will share the following basic features:

- on/off switch

- output channels

- power source – usually a 6 or 9 volt battery

- intensity controls for each output

- frequency controls – two frequency range settings: 0 to 100 and 10 to 999 Hz (there is often a switch that changes the output by a factor of 10, changing it to a TENS machine)

- dense–disperse controls

- Loc–Needle–Stimulation treatment and location switch.

Lee (2012) clarifies the confusion surrounding the use of red and black leads on EA machines. As an alternating current (AC) does not have permanent positive or negative polarities, and therefore is constantly changing from positive to negative, it doesn't matter which way round the leads are placed.

Figure 12.5 is a standard EA machine with labels.

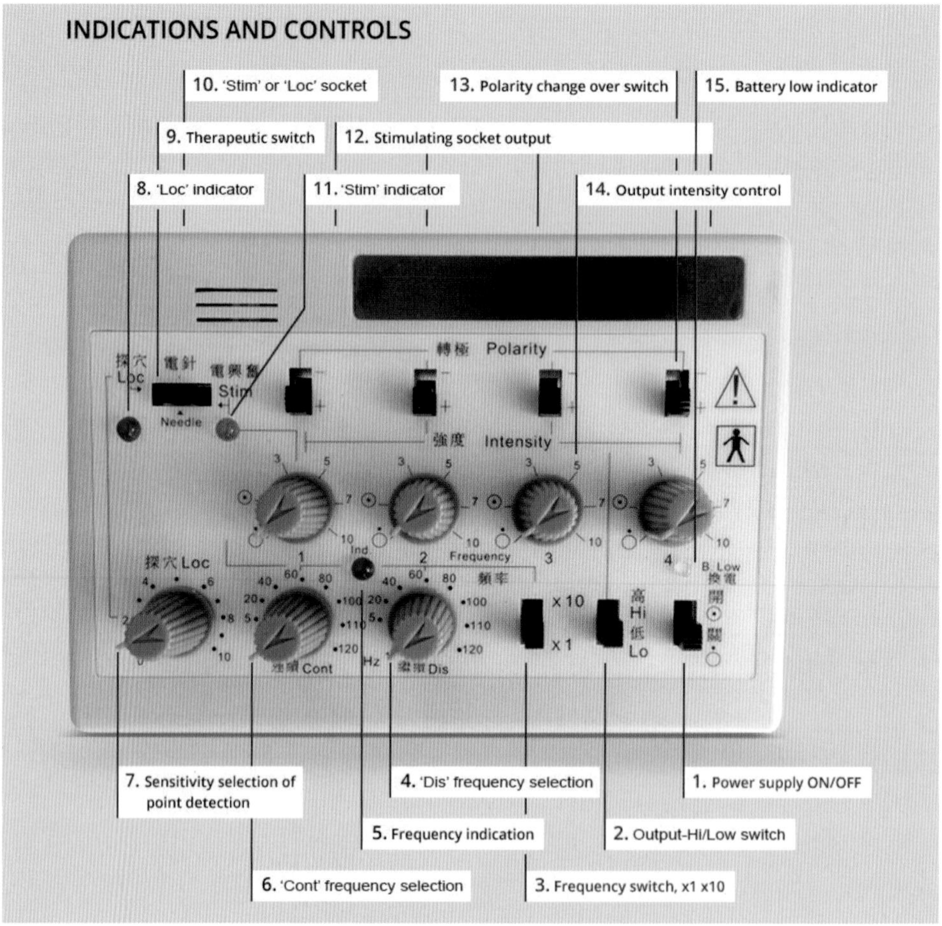

Figure 12.5 A standard EA machine

Needle placement for EA treatment

EA can be provided on a number of acupuncture points and meridians, including the classical bilateral acupuncture points, spinal acupuncture points and myofascial meridians. While treating the joints with EA, a needle pair should cross the joint or with as much of the joint as possible between them, so that the patient can experience a sensation of electrical current travelling through the affected joint.

The protocols suggested are just some basic guidelines and should be treated as such. Once the basic principle has been grasped and experience and confidence developed in using EA, then one can apply the basic ideas, theories and protocols to a variety of conditions.

Note: An electric current does not always flow directly from point A to point B in a straight line, because it has a tendency to move through the path of least resistance.

Frequency of treatment

Frequency of treatment in the West is often dictated by time and money, usually with treatment weekly and sometimes twice weekly. Typically there should be an improvement after 4–6 treatments, but sometimes more sessions are required. If treating an ongoing problem such as osteoarthritis, then top-up treatment every few months will be required.

Technique descriptions

In this section we show a selection of EA techniques for joints and muscles. In practice, EA can be used on any major muscle within the body as long as you follow the protocols for needle placement; see Chapter 11 for additional EA techniques.

Plastic-handled needles as shown in the photos in this section are used for demonstration purposes and should not be used for actual EA treatments. The coloured dotted lines represent the flow of current between two needles, which is where a single output would be connected from the EA machine. However, these are only suggestions and there is no wrong or right way.

Low back pain

Obviously, low back pain can have a multitude of sources. Needling depth varies according to the patient's size. Often deep needling is necessary to affect the deep stabilizing muscles of the lumbar spine using a .50 or .75 needle.

In the photo below the huatuojiaji points (lateral to the lower border of each spinous process) of L1 and L5 have been used, with the green and yellow dots representing the flow of current between L1 and L5. The blue and red dots are connected to the other points, which are trigger points in the quadratus lumborum.

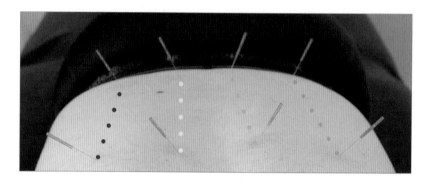

Achilles tendon

The Achilles tendon is covered in depth in Chapter 13. A simple protocol which can be effective is to use a four-needle cross-pattern technique. Two needles are inserted near the insertion of the Achilles and the other pair are inserted superiorly to these, still within the Achilles tendon. The photo below simply shows that the needles are connected diagonally, with one pair connected to the inferior medial needle and the other to the superior lateral needle, and vice versa. The red and yellow dotted lines represent the current flowing through the Achilles.

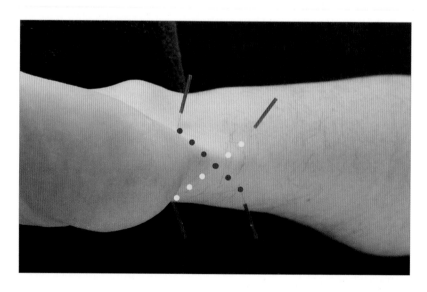

Inversion sprain

The following points are used:

- Gallbladder 40 (anterior and inferior to the external malleolus, in the depression on the lateral side of the tendon of m. extensor digitorum longus) is paired with non-acupuncture points anterior to the lateral malleolus between the tibialis anterior tendon, shown with the red dotted line in the photo below.

- Stomach 41 (in the depression at the midpoint of the transverse crease of the ankle between the tendons m. extensor hallucis longus and digitorum longus) is paired with Bladder 60 (midway between the high point of the outer ankle bone and the Achilles tendon), shown with the yellow dotted line in the photo.

This creates a cross-pattern technique across the common ligaments often involved in inversion sprains.

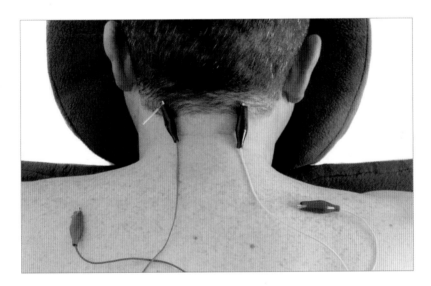

Knee pain

The following points are used often with osteoarthritis patients:

- eyes of the knee (a pair of points in the two depressions, medial and lateral to the patellar ligament, locating the point with the knee flexed)

- Spleen 10

- Stomach 33/34.

Create a cross-pattern with the medial eye of the knee point connected to Spleen 10 with the other eye of the knee point to Stomach 33/34. The red and yellow dots in the photo below show the current passing through the knee.

Additional points can be used to pass any further current through the knee for a greater effect, essentially anterior to posterior and medial to lateral. For example:

- From Liver 8 to a point of the lateral side anterior to the hamstring tendon.

- From Bladder 40 to a point superior to the quadriceps tendon.

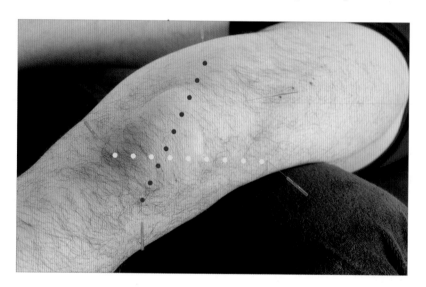

Hip pain

Needle the following points:

- Gallbladder 30 or a trigger point in the piriformis to a trigger point in the tensor fasciae latae.

- A trigger point below the anterior superior iliac spine (origin of TFL) to a trigger point located inferior to the greater trochanter on or near Gallbladder 31 in the iliotibial band or near vastus lateralis. The red and yellow dots in the photo below represent the flow of current between the points described.

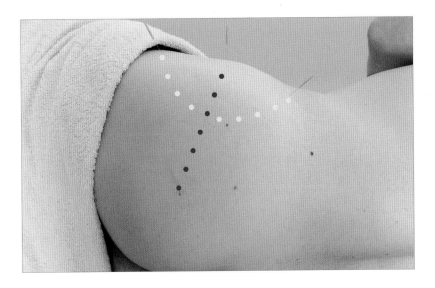

Knuckle and finger joints

Use small needles for this procedure. If in the early stages of trigger finger, then the hand will have to be palm face-up; otherwise it is preferable for the palm to be face down. Simply needle either proximal interphalangeal joints or the metacarpophalangeal joints with a needle inserted either side of the joint, with EA then applied, which passes through the joint. Ensure that the needles are not touching, as this will create a short circuit. You can use cotton wool between the needles to stop this from happening.

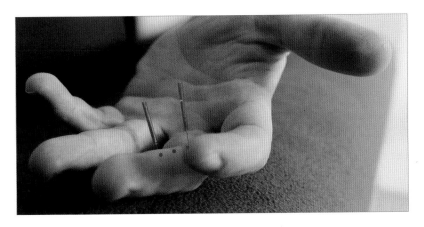

Neck pain

Needle the following points:

- Bladder 10 (in the depression on the lateral aspect of muscle trapezius below the hairline) to a trigger point in the upper trapezius. Other points can be substituted.

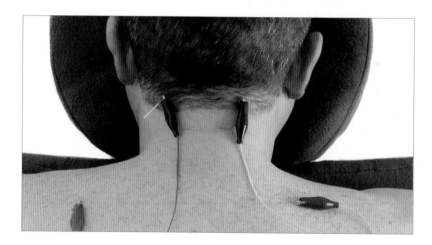

Carpal tunnel

Needle the following points:

- Pericardium 8 (in the centre of the palm, between the second and third metacarpal bones) to Pericardium 5 (between the tendons of m. palmaris longus and m. flexor carpi radialis), shown with the yellow dotted line in the photo below.

- Large Intestine 5 (in the anatomical snuffbox, in the depression between the tendons extensor pollicis longus and brevis) to Small Intestine 4 (ulnar aspect of the palm, in the depression between the fifth metacarpal bone and hamate bone), shown with the red dotted line in the photo.

In addition, palpate for trigger points in the flexor muscles and screen for thoracic outlet syndrome or cervical dysfunction.

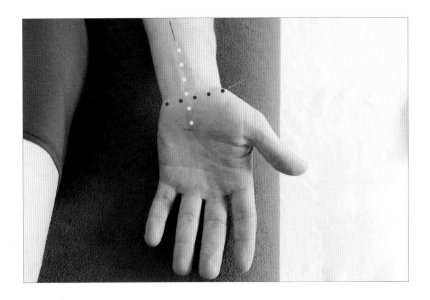

References

Ahn, A.C., Colbert, A.P., Anderson, B.J., *et al.* (2008) 'Electrical properties of acupuncture points and meridians: a systematic review.' *Bioelectromagnetics 29*, 4, 245–256.

Baek, Y.H., Yang, H.I., and Park, D.S. (2005) 'Analgesic effect of electroacupuncture on inflammatory pain in the rat model of collagen-induced arthritis: mediation by cholinergic and serotonergic receptors.' *Brain Research 1057*, 1, 181–185.

Cagnie, B., Dewitte, V., Barbe, T., Timmermans, F., Delrue, N., and Meeus, M. (2013) 'Physiologic effects of dry needling.' *Current Pain and Headache Reports 17*, 8, 1–8.

Cameron, M.H. (2012) *Physical Agents in Rehabilitation: From Research to Practice.* New York: Elsevier Health Sciences.

Chen, X.H., and Han, J.S. (1992) 'Analgesia induced by electroacupuncture of different frequencies is mediated by different types of opioid receptors: another cross-tolerance study.' *Behavioural Brain Research 47*, 2, 143–149.

Chung, J.M., Fang, Z.R., Hori, Y., Lee, K.H., and Willis, W.D. (1984) 'Prolonged inhibition of primate spinothalamic tract cells by peripheral nerve stimulation.' *Pain 19*, 3, 259–275.

Cummings, M. (2011) 'Safety aspects of electroacupuncture.' *Acupunct. Med. 29*, 2, 83–85.

Curatolo, M., Arendt-Nielsen, L., and Petersen-Felix, S. (2006) 'Central hypersensitivity in chronic pain: mechanisms and clinical implications.' *Phys. Med. Rehabil. Clin. N. Am. 17*, 2, 287–302.

Dharmananda, S. (2002) *Electro-acupuncture.* Institute for Traditional Medicine. Available at www.itmonline.org/arts/electro.htm, accessed on 27 July 2015.

Garrison, F.H. (1921) *An Introduction to the History of Medicine c. 2.* Philadelphia and London: W.B. Saunders.

Gildenberg, P.L. (2006) 'History of electrical neuromodulation for chronic pain.' *Pain Medicine 7*, s1, S7–S13.

Guo, H.F., Tian, J., Wang, X., Fang, Y., Hou, Y., and Han, J. (1996) 'Brain substrates activated by electroacupuncture of different frequencies (I): comparative study on the expression of oncogene c-fos and genes coding for three opioid peptides.' *Molecular Brain Research* *43*, 1, 157–166.

Han, J.S. (2003) 'Acupuncture: neuropeptide release produced by electrical stimulation of different frequencies.' *Trends in Neurosciences 26*, 1, 17–22.

Han, J.S. (2004) 'Acupuncture and endorphins.' *Neuroscience Letters 361*, 1, 258–261.

Han, Z., Jiang, Y.H., Wan, Y., Wang, Y., Chang, J.K., and Han, J.S. (1999) 'Endomorphin-1 mediates 2 Hz but not 100 Hz electroacupuncture analgesia in the rat.' *Neuroscience Letters 274*, 2, 75–78.

Hsieh, C.L., Kuo, C.C., Chen, Y.S., *et al.* (2000) 'Analgesic effect of electric stimulation of peripheral nerves with different electric frequencies using the formalin test.' *American Journal of Chinese Medicine 28*, 2, 291–299.

Huang, C., Li, H.T., Shi, Y.S., Han, J.S., and Wan, Y. (2004) 'Ketamine potentiates the effect of electroacupuncture on mechanical allodynia in a rat model of neuropathic pain.' *Neuroscience Letters 368*, 3, 327–331.

Kim, S.K., Park, J.H., Bae, S.J., *et al.* (2005) 'Effects of electroacupuncture on cold allodynia in a rat model of neuropathic pain: mediation by spinal adrenergic and serotonergic receptors.' *Experimental Neurology 195*, 2, 430–436.

Lee, B.Y., LaRiccia, P.J., and Newberg, A.B. (2004a) 'Acupuncture in theory and practice part 1: theoretical basis and physiologic effects.' *Hospital Physician 40*, 4, 11–18.

Lee, B.Y., LaRiccia, P.J., and Newberg, A.B. (2004b) 'Acupuncture in theory and practice part 2: clinical indications, efficacy, and safety.' *Hospital Physician 40*, 5, 33–38.

Lee, S. (2012) 'Electroacupuncture for the treatment of musculoskeletal conditions.' *Journal of Chinese Medicine 99*, 14–24.

Leung, A., Khadivi, B., Duann, J.R., Cho, Z.H., and Yaksh, T. (2005) 'The effect of Ting point (tendinomuscular meridians) electroacupuncture on thermal pain: a model for studying the neuronal mechanism of acupuncture analgesia.' *Journal of Alternative & Complementary Medicine 11*, 4, 653–661.

Leung, L. (2012) 'Neurophysiological basis of acupuncture-induced analgesia – an updated review.' *J. Acupunct. Meridian Stud. 5*, 6, 261–270.

Lianfang, H.E. (1987) 'Involvement of endogenous opioid peptides in acupuncture analgesia.' *Pain 31*, 1, 99–121.

Lin, J.G., and Chen, W.L. (2008) 'Acupuncture analgesia: a review of its mechanisms of actions.' *American Journal of Chinese Medicine 36*, 4, 635–645.

MacPherson, H., Scullion, A., Thomas, K.J., and Walters, S. (2004) 'Patient reports of adverse events associated with acupuncture treatment: a prospective national survey.' *Quality and Safety in Health Care 13*, 5, 349–355.

Mayer, D.J., Price, D.D., and Rafii, A. (1977) 'Antagonism of acupuncture analgesia in man by the narcotic antagonist naloxone.' *Brain Research 121*, 2, 368–372.

Mayor, D.F. (2007a) 'Electroacupuncture: an introduction and its use for peripheral facial paralysis.' *Journal of Chinese Medicine 84*, 52–63.

Mayor, D.F. (ed.) (2007b) *Electroacupuncture: A Practical Manual and Resource.* New York: Elsevier Health Sciences. Companion website available at www.electroacupunctureknowledge. com, accessed on 27 July 2015.

Melzack, R., and Wall, P.D. (1967) 'Pain mechanisms: a new theory.' *Survey of Anesthesiology 11*, 2, 89–90.

Noordergraaf, A., and Silage, D. (1973) 'Electroacupuncture.' *IEEE Transactions on Biomedical Engineering 5*, 364–366.

Okada, K., and Kawakita, K. (2009) 'Analgesic action of acupuncture and moxibustion: a review of unique approaches in Japan.' *Evidence-Based Complementary and Alternative Medicine 6*, 1, 11–17.

Paraskevaidis, S., Mochlas, S., Hadjimiltiadis, S., and Louridas, G. (1999) 'Intermittent P wave sensing in a patient with DDD pacemaker.' *Pacing and Clinical Electrophysiology 22*, 4, 689–690.

Pomeranz, B., and Chiu, D. (1976) 'Naloxone blockade of acupuncture analgesia: endorphin implicated.' *Life Sciences 19*, 11, 1757–1762.

Pomeranz, B., and Paley, D. (1979) 'Electroacupuncture hypalgesia is mediated by afferent nerve impulses: an electrophysiological study in mice.' *Experimental Neurology 66*, 2, 398–402.

Pomeranz, B., Cheng, R., and Law, P. (1977) 'Acupuncture reduces electrophysiological and behavioral responses to noxious stimuli: pituitary is implicated.' *Experimental Neurology 54*, 1, 172–178.

Pyne, D., and Shenker, N.G. (2008) 'Demystifying acupuncture.' *Rheumatology 47*, 8, 1132–1136.

Silvério-Lopes, S. (2011) 'Electroacupuncture and stimulatory frequencies for analgesia: acupuncture, concepts and physiology.' *Rijeka (Croatia): In Tech*, 69–90. Available at http://cdn.intechopen.com/pdfs-wm/21304.pdf, accessed on 27 July 2015.

Takagi, J., and Yonehara, N. (1998) 'Serotonin receptor subtypes involved in modulation of electrical acupuncture.' *Japanese Journal of Pharmacology 78*, 4, 511–514.

Toda, K. (2002) 'Afferent Nerve Characteristics During Acupuncture Stimulation.' In A. Sato, P. Li and J.L. Campbell (eds) *Acupuncture – Is There a Physiological Basis?* International Congress Series Vol. 1238. New York: Elsevier.

Tsai, H.-Y., Chen, Y.-F., and Lin, J.-G. (1989) 'Effect of electroacupuncture analgesia on serotoninergic neurons in rat central nervous system.' *Chin. Pharmacol. J. 41*, 123–126.

Walsh, S., and Berry, K. (2010) 'Electroacupuncture and TENS: putting theory into practice.' *Journal of Chinese Medicine 92*, 46–58.

Woolf, C.J. (1984) 'Transcutaneous and Implanted Nerve Stimulation.' In P.D. Wall and R. Melzack (eds) *Textbook of Pain*. Edinburgh: Churchill Livingstone.

World Health Organization (1999) *Guidelines on Basic Training and Safety in Acupuncture.* Available at http://whqlibdoc.who.int/hq/1999/WHO_EDM_TRM_99.1.pdf, accessed on 22 July 2015.

Yang, J., Yang, Y., Chen, J.M., Liu, W.Y., Wang, C.H., and Lin, B.C. (2007) 'Effect of oxytocin on acupuncture analgesia in the rat.' *Neuropeptides 41*, 5, 285–292.

Yoo, Y.C., Oh, J.H., Kwon, T.D., Lee, Y.K., and Bai, S.J. (2011) 'Analgesic mechanism of electroacupuncture in an arthritic pain model of rats: a neurotransmitter study.' *Yonsei Medical Journal 52*, 6, 1016–1021.

Zhang, R.X., Liu, B., Qiao, J.T., *et al.* (2005a) 'Electroacupuncture suppresses spinal expression of neurokinin-1 receptors induced by persistent inflammation in rats.' *Neuroscience Letters 384*, 3, 339–343.

Zhang, R.X., Wang, L., Wang, X., Ren, K., Berman, B.M., and Lao, L. (2005b) 'Electroacupuncture combined with MK-801 prolongs anti-hyperalgesia in rats with peripheral inflammation.' *Pharmacology Biochemistry and Behavior 81*, 1, 146–151.

Zhao, Z.Q. (2008) 'Neural mechanism underlying acupuncture analgesia.' *Progress in Neurobiology 85*, 4, 355–375.

Chapter 13

Tendinopathy and Tendon Techniques

The term 'tendinopathy' describes a variety of disorders of tendon structure that result in significant pain and dysfunction at all ages and activity levels. Prior to the 1990s, pain arising from tendons was referred to as tendinitis, implying that inflammation was responsible for the pathological process initially recognized by Puddu and others in the 1970s. In more recent studies, and as histological tendinopathy data increased, it was found that chronic tendinopathy had a distinct lack of acute inflammatory cells, and as this became increasingly recognized the term tendinitis was discouraged as a diagnosis (Rees, Stride and Scott 2013). Thus the term tendinopathy has replaced the terms 'tendinosis' and 'tendinitis' (or 'tendonitis') due to degenerative change but no inflammation being found in histopathological examination (Xu and Murrell 2008). However, Rees *et al.* (2013) consider that categorizing chronic tendinopathy as entirely non-inflammatory is an oversimplification to the point of being misleading.

Tendinopathy includes varying conditions which can be further classified, including disorders of the connective tissue (paratendinitis) or synovial tendon sheath (tenosynovitis), insertional tendinopathy, tendon rupture pathologies at the enthesis (insertion), and pathologies of the core tendon itself (Speed 2015).

Tendinopathy can occur in almost any major tendon. Some common clinical examples include supraspinatus, rotator cuff, plantar fascia, Achilles tendon, patellar tendon, and lateral and medial epicondyle. There is an increased incidence with age, male gender and obesity. There is also an association between tendinopathy and hormone replacement therapy and oral contraceptives in women.

Lack of understanding of this condition has led to speculation about efficient treatment options. There are a wide range of possible options including conservative (manual therapy and exercise prescription), pharmacological and surgical options. Currently there is no gold standard for treatment (Xu and Murrell 2008). The multitude of approaches to management of a clinical problem suggests either that it is quite responsive to intervention or that the optimal approaches have yet to be identified.

Conservative measures include rest, activity modification, non-steroidal anti-inflammatory medications, manual therapy and corticosteroid injections. Eccentric exercises, involving the motion of an active muscle while it is lengthening under load, are often used as part of a conservative programme and are a way of promoting collagen fibre cross-linkage, creating a remodelling process. Success is limited due to patient compliance; and whilst the effectiveness of exercise is established, the uptake of and adherence to exercise is poor. Deep friction massage and myofascial techniques have been shown to stimulate fibroblast proliferation, leading to collagen synthesis that may promote healing by replacing degenerative tissue with a stronger and more functional tissue.

There is substantial evidence that corticosteroids can be effective at relieving pain in chronic tendinopathy, reducing swelling and improving function in the short term, although at the expense of greater risk of long-term recurrence. The issues relating to corticosteroid injection are therefore less that they do not work, but more that the benefits are generally short term, and that there is the potential for weakening the structural integrity of tendons in the long term.

Normal tendon function and structure

Tendons are anatomic structures between muscles and bones that transmit the force created in muscle to bone and make joint movement possible. During high-impact exercise activities, very high loads are placed on tendons, and those such as the Achilles are at the highest risk for rupture if tension is applied quickly and obliquely (racket sports being one such example). Tendons are capable of handling high loads, and studies have shown that they have the ability to handle up to ten times a human's bodyweight during stress tests to meet this demand (Khan 2003).

The basic elements of tendon are collagen bundles, cells and ground substance or extracellular matrix, a viscous substance rich in proteoglycans. Collagen provides tendons with tensile strength; ground substance provides structural support for the collagen fibres and regulates the extracellular assembly of procollagen into mature collagen.

Within the extracellular matrix network, tenoblasts and tenocytes constitute about 90–95 per cent of the cellular elements of tendons. Tenoblasts are immature tendon cells. As they mature, tenoblasts become elongated and transform into tenocytes. The remaining 5–10 per cent of the cellular elements of tendons consists of chondrocytes at the bone attachment and insertion sites, synovial cells of the tendon sheath, and vascular cells, including capillary endothelial cells and the smooth muscle cells of arterioles (Sharma and Maffulli 2005).

Collagen is arranged in hierarchical levels of increasing complexity and are mainly oriented longitudinally, but fibres can also run transversely and horizontally, forming spirals and plaits. The matrix has tight bundles of long strands of type I collagen, which give the tendon its inherent strength. Most of the fibres are arranged parallel to the direction of force (Cook, Khan and Purdam 2002).

The entire tendon is covered by the epitenon, a fine, loose connective tissue sheath containing the vascular, lymphatic and nerve supply. More superficially, the epitenon is surrounded by paratenon, a loose areolar connective tissue consisting essentially of type I and type III collagen fibrils, some elastic fibrils and an inner lining of synovial cells. Together, the paratenon and epitenon are sometimes called the peritendon. The Achilles peritendon does not have a synovial layer found in hand and wrist tendons (Cook *et al.* 2002).

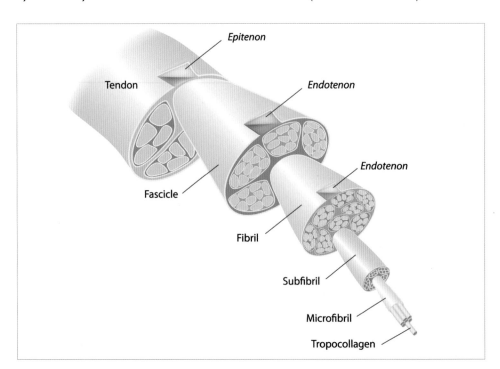

Figure 13.1 The tendon structure

There are two important junctions in tendons, the myotendinous and osteotendinous junctions. The myotendinous junction is a highly specialized anatomic region in the muscle–tendon unit where tension generated by muscle fibres is transmitted to the tendon (Charvet, Ruggiero and Le Guellec 2012). The myotendinous junction is the weakest point of the muscle–tendon unit. The osteotendinous junction is where the tendon inserts into a bone. This junction is where the tendon transmits the force into a rigid bone. These interfaces also serve to dissipate stress between soft tissue and bone (Khan 2003).

Both intrinsic systems and extrinsic systems provide the main blood supply for tendons, but this varies from tendon to tendon. The intrinsic system includes both the myotendinous junction and the osteotendinous junction. The extrinsic system is supplied via the paratenon or the synovial sheath. The blood supply from the osteotendinous junction is minimal and limited to the local site of tendon insertion. The myotendinous junction is richer in its supply than the osteotendinous junction (Sharma and Maffulli 2005).

Tendons have an extremely well-developed anaerobic capacity and low metabolic rate, which allows them to sustain high loads for long periods. This has the biological advantage of avoiding ischaemia and early necrosis in these vital structures.

The oxygen consumption by tendons and ligaments is significantly lower than that of skeletal muscle, often as much as 7.5 times lower, a major disadvantage when factoring tendons' slow healing times. In general, tendon blood flow declines with increasing age and mechanical loading. Given that tendons require approximately 100 days to synthesize the main structural proteins, frequent microtrauma during chronic and excessive loading may not allow sufficient time for tendon repair. Tendon strength is directly correlated with the collagen amount and is therefore critical in correct functioning.

Different tendons have different properties, with larger tendons being able to withstand larger forces, whilst longer tendons are able to elongate further before fibril disruption occurs. Tendons have high mechanical strength and low elasticity. However, these properties are only maintained when the tendon is elongated, and it has weak resistance to compressive and shear forces (Selvanetti, Cipolla and Puddu 1997).

Tendon failure

Tendons of certain anatomical locations are more susceptible in individuals who are older, heavier and male in those genetically predisposed to tendinopathy. Active repair of fatigue damage must occur, or tendons would weaken and eventually rupture; however, this is an extremely fine balance between extracellular matrix (ECM) production and degradation. One current hypothesis is that tendinopathy occurs when tendon cells experience a large amount of repetitive load (volume, intensity and frequency), resulting in various failed healing responses as the demands on the tendon are higher than can be managed adequately with the normal healing response. Xu and Murrell (2008) describe four cornerstones of tendon histopathology:

1. cellular activation and increase in cell numbers

2. increase in ground substance

3. collagen disarray

4. neovascularization.

Cook and Purdam (2009) propose that there is a continuum of tendon pathology which has three stages: reactive tendinopathy, tendon disrepair (failed healing) and degenerative tendinopathy. They maintain that there is continuity throughout the different stages.

The reactive stage is a short-term adaptation to overload that thickens the tendon, reduces stress and increases stiffness. This stage can be reverted to normal if the overload is sufficiently reduced or if there is sufficient time between loading sessions. Therefore, assessment and modification of the intensity, duration, frequency and type of load are the keys of the clinical intervention (Marchand, O'Shaughnessy and Descarreaux 2014).

Tendon disrepair describes the failed attempt at tendon healing. There may be an increase in vascularity and associated neuronal ingrowth. There is a marked increase in proteoglycan and collagen production. The increase in proteoglycans results in separation of the collagen and disorganization of the matrix accompanied with neurovascularity of the tendon. The frequency, volume and length of time over which load has been applied seem to be important variables in predicting the degree of reversibility, which is still possible with load management (Marchand *et al.* 2014).

The final stage of degenerative tendinopathy sees a further disruption of collagen, widespread cell death and extensive ingrowth of neovessels and

Dry Needling for Manual Therapists

nerves into the tendon substance, leading to an essentially irreversible stage of pathology (McCreesh and Lewis 2013).

The Cook and Purdam (2009) model is widely supported, though the optimal intervention for each stage of pathology is still unknown. There are many cases where structure does not parallel pain, therefore the use of imaging is useful. Neal and Longbottom (2012) suggest that the gold standard should be diagnostic confirmation by ultrasound because the use of ultrasound scanning is recommended as a way of clinically differentiating between the phases, with neovessels and a hyperechoic appearance of collagen fibres being markers of degenerative pathology.

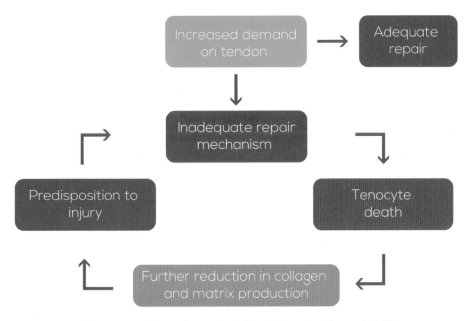

Figure 13.2 The tendon cycle (adapted from Leadbetter 1992)

Whilst pain is a driving factor for patients presenting with tendinopathy, and the eradication of pain often being the clinical goal, determining the source of pain is difficult. Subjective pain and the correlation of symptoms are often mismatched. Current theories suggest that the pain arises from biochemical irritants, peritendinous tissues or neurovascular ingrowth (McCreesh and Lewis 2013). For example, glutamate, a well-known neurotransmitter and very potent modulator of pain in the central nervous system, is found in high levels in painful tendons but not in normal tendons (Alfredson and Cook 2007).

Tendon underload

Arnoczky, Lavagnino and Egerbacher (2007) presented an argument for the mechanobiological under-stimulation of tendon cells, secondary to microtrauma and isolated collagen fibril damage, as a predisposing factor for the pathological changes found in tendinopathy. In this proposal, stress deprivation (lack of loading) leads to upregulation of collagenase expression and apoptosis of tendon cells, leading to decreased structural and mechanical properties and leaving the tendon capacity unable to tolerate load. This model is useful when considering tendinopathy in sedentary patient populations and also active populations who have had a period of rest (off-season or through injury) and then return to active participation in their chosen sport or activity.

Obesity

Obesity is a worldwide epidemic, and one of the major public health problems in Western countries. Obesity is a well-recognized risk factor for cardiovascular diseases but is also a factor in increased susceptibility to musculoskeletal disorders. It is a widely held belief that tendinopathy is typically due to tendon overload; however, studies suggest that obesity is a risk factor for tendinopathy and that obese patients often have a poor clinical outcome both in rehabilitation and surgical procedures. There may be both mechanical and biochemical reasons for this increased risk. The two hypotheses for the two different mechanisms are the increased yield on the load-bearing tendons and the biochemical alterations attributed to systemic dysmetabolic factors (Nantel, Mathieu and Prince 2011).

Obese individuals have also been shown to modify the force alignment and consequently the distribution of forces at the knee during weight-bearing. In adults, an increased bodyweight leads to major modifications in the gait pattern. Obese individuals have been shown to walk with a shorter step length, lower cadence and velocity, a decrease in the duration of the simple support phase and an increased double support phase. The increase in load when combined with shear and compressive forces may increase susceptibility to tendinopathy (Nantel *et al.* 2011).

Typically, obese patients have a chronic low-grade inflammatory state. As a consequence, Abate (2014, p.37) claims that 'the release of profibrotic factors, such as TGF-β, is reduced, and this may have a detrimental effect on tendon healing, especially if the production of type I and III collagen is also reduced. The main histopathologic findings are a relative paucity of small collagen fibrils, expression of an impaired remodelling process, deposition of lipid droplets which can abut to tendolipomatosis, and a disorganized architecture in the tension regions.' Both load-bearing and non-load-bearing tendons can be affected. Because thin fibres confer greater elasticity to tendons, their relative scarcity could be responsible for increased stiffness and microruptures as a consequence of excessive loads (Abate 2014).

Generally, obese patients are encouraged to participate in some form of physical activity to reduce weight and associated health risks. However, this should be graded, and attention to weight-bearing activities should be introduced gradually or substituted for non-weight-bearing activities because obese patients may have tendons with subclinical damage, and overload can easily reach the symptomatic threshold, signalling the start of tendinopathy and possibly preventing any further physical activity.

Use of acupuncture

Borchers, Krey and McCamey (2015) conducted a systemic review on tendon needling for treatment of tendinopathy and concluded that tendon needling improves patient-reported outcome measures in patients. However, only four studies met the inclusion criteria. This highlights the need for high-quality research-based evidence to determine acupuncture's potential use in treating tendinopathies.

Neal and Longbottom (2012, p.346) echo these findings: 'We would suggest that there is a small but high quality contingent of evidence supporting the theory that acupuncture may be able to influence tendon healing by increasing blood flow via local vasodilation and increasing collagen proliferation. These effects are most likely a result of an increase of the neuropeptide CGRP from sensory nerve endings and an increase in mechanical signalling through the extracellular matrix respectively.' However, the absence of evidence does not mean that acupuncture is unable to effect tendon healing – it just hasn't been proven effective or ineffective yet.

It is now well documented that acupuncture performed at local sites releases powerful vasodilators, but more research in healthy and pathological human tendon tissue would be required to further support this theory. Kubo *et al.* (2010) found that acupuncture on tendons increased the blood volume and oxygen saturation of the tendon and that this was maintained post-acupuncture. By increasing blood flow, oxygenation and tissue healing can occur in the tendon. Supporting the intrinsic healing of tendons (through acupuncture or other means) will result in better biomechanical remodelling of the tendon.

When considering Cook and Purdam's (2009) tendinopathy continuum model, it is important to establish the effects of acupuncture's role in treating tendinopathies and to establish the stage or stages at which the most beneficial effects may be achieved.

De Almeida *et al.* (2014) hypothesized that acupuncture can modulate both anti-inflammatory (AI) and mechanotransduction (MT) molecular pathways. The modulation of these pathways can increase type I collagen synthesis and subsequent reorganization, allowing an increase in the load-bearing capacity of the tendon.

The addition of electroacupuncture to treatment protocols may have an additional benefit. De Almeida, De Freitas and De Oliveira (2015) found that when using EA it resulted in an increase in collagen fibril diameter and reorganization potential for increased synthesis and reorganization of type I collagen, which is the major tendon structural component (approximately 95% of the total collagen). Inoue *et al.* (2015, p.60) concluded: 'Our key findings were that the application of EA [electroacupuncture] to a tendon rupture model increased total cell counts, TGF-β1 and b-FGF positive cell counts, and also the mechanical strength of repaired tendon compared with control groups receiving MA [manual acupuncture] or no treatment.' Both of these were animal studies, and need to be replicated in human studies, both healthy and pathological, to confirm the hypothesis.

There is further speculation that acupuncture may result in reduction in mechanical hypersensitivity through effects on neurotransmitters, neurotrophin expression and neuromodulation (Speed 2015).

The use of segmental acupuncture may be of further benefit to tendon healing. Acupuncture when applied segmentally can inhibit the pre-synaptic release of glutamate, a nociceptive neurotransmitter consistently seen in degenerative tendons (Zhao 2008).

It is well documented that glutamate and its receptors play a pivotal role in the spinal transmission of nociceptive information and central sensitization in physiological and pathological conditions. EA may further enhance this effect when applied segmentally.

Key points

- Currently only small, though high-quality, studies have been carried out to support acupuncture for tendon healing.

- Vasodilators are released when needling local points and further increased by choosing points in or near myotendinous and osteotendinous junctions.

- Acupuncture results in increased collagen reorganization.

- The above points lead to reduced pain and increased loading capacity.

- Periosteal pecking may be beneficial (see below).

- Acupuncture results in reduction in central sensitization.

- EA may have significant benefit over MA.

- Combining acupuncture into manual therapy and exercise therapy may result in improved patient outcome compared with acupuncture as a stand-alone therapy.

Possible acupuncture protocols

Acupuncture can be used as a stand-alone therapy or as a component of a combination of therapies. There is no standard acupuncture treatment for tendinopathy; rather, there are a number of possibilities. These may include the following:

- crossing-pattern technique – using four needles across a joint

- selecting points near myotendinous and osteotendinous junctions

- direct needling of tendon

- thread needling along tendon

- use of local, distal and adjacent TCM points (yuan, jing well, shu stream, he sea)

- layering effect (local, supraspinal and segmental points)

- periosteal pecking

- surrounding dragon technique (needle circling)

- use of EA.

Periosteal pecking

Periosteal pecking (sometimes referred to as osteoacupuncture) is a form of acupuncture in which the tip of the needle contacts the periosteum. When one hits the bone with the tip of the needle, the needle is used to peck the bone. The same place of periosteum is not pecked repeatedly but the tip is moved around a small distance to peck a larger area (Mann 2000). The area that is pecked is typically around 0.25–0.5 inches in diameter, and is pecked 2–4 times per second for between 10 and 30 seconds. Patients usually experience some deqi, and the needles are left in for between 10 and 30 minutes without further stimulation (unless EA is applied).

The success of periosteal pecking in comparison with other modalities warrants further investigation, especially when combined with manual acupuncture or electroacupuncture. It seems plausible that combining periosteal pecking, MA and EA will have increased benefits. In an experimental study in healthy volunteers, electrical stimulation of the periosteum was superior to stimulation of musculature and skin in alleviating pain originating from the periosteum and musculature (Hansson, Carlsson and Olsson 2008).

The technique can be painful, as the periosteum has nociceptive nerve endings, making it very sensitive to stimulation. Therefore consideration of toleration of pain levels versus clinical outcome may be required when considering using this technique.

Clinical trials and literature on the use of periosteal pecking are sparse, but the treatment has been used in the treatment of shin splints, osteoarthritis of the knee and hip, cervical disorders and other MSK conditions.

Techniques

Achilles tendon

The Achilles tendon attaches the posterior calf muscles – the gastrocnemius and soleus – to the calcaneus. Its action is to actively plantar flex the ankle, and to resist dorsiflexion. There is a bursa interposed between the anterior surface of the tendon and the surface of the calcaneus.

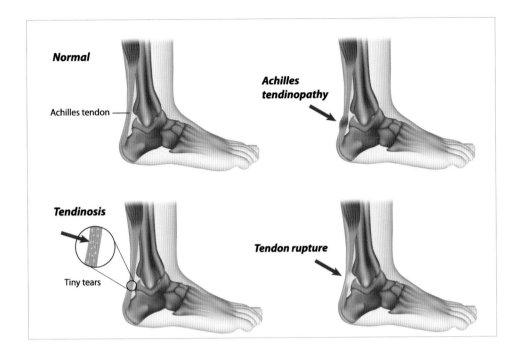

Figure 13.3 Achilles tendon problems

Fahlström *et al.* (2003) found that Achilles tendinopathy accounts for 6–17 per cent of all running injuries among recreational runners, and the incidence is higher with older age and male gender. The peak age for Achilles rupture is 30–40, when degenerative changes and continued or occasional high stress from sports combine.

There are two main tendinopathies – mid-portion Achilles tendinopathy and insertional tendinopathy, with mid-portion being more frequent. The mid-portion tendinopathy is roughly 1–2.5 inches above the insertion point of the Achilles tendon on the calcaneus and is an area of diminished blood supply, leaving it susceptible to injury. Insertional tendinopathy affects the insertion of the tendon on the calcaneus, comprising around 25 per cent of cases compared with 75 per cent of cases of mid-portion tendinopathy (BMJ 2012).

Generally, the initial treatment consists of a multifactorial approach that may include a combination of rest (complete or modified activity), medication (NSAIDs, corticosteroids), orthotic treatment (heel lift, change of shoes, corrections of malalignments), stretching and strength training. If conservative treatment fails, surgical treatment is instituted (Alfredson and Cook 2007).

Herringbone technique

For mid-portion Achilles tendinopathy, the herringbone technique is recommended. This method has recently been adopted by acupuncturists and is referred to as the herringbone technique because of its appearance. The configuration is achieved by inserting needles vertically, medially and laterally (i.e. parallel) to the tendon. The herringbone technique is mainly used in the Achilles tendon because of its accessibility, and is taught on acupuncture courses (Kishmishian, Selfe and Richards 2012). A possible standardization of the technique is to have four needles for each surface (vertically, medially and laterally) and equal distance from each other. The needle penetrates the tendon to a depth of around 0.2 inches (though measurements only serve as a guide, as there are differences from patient to patient). Additional needling of the soleus and gatrocnemius (posterior chain) may be beneficial, points such as Bladder 58, 57, 56 and 55, inner/outer bladder points and huatuojiaji points. EA can be applied in a cross-pattern and along the vertical portion of the tendon using an additional pair.

For insertional tendinopathy, the herringbone technique can be used with the addition of periosteal pecking into the calcaneal insertion.

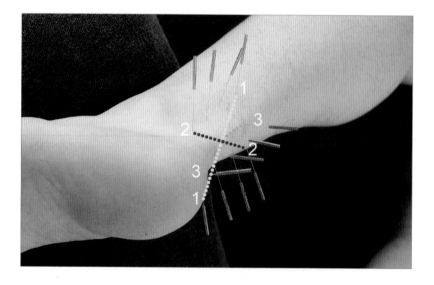

Percutaneous tenotomy and acupuncture scraping technique

Several new treatments have been developed in an attempt to stimulate tissue regeneration. One of these treatments is a percutaneous needle tenotomy, in which the area of tendinopathy is repetitively fenestrated with a needle to disrupt tendinopathic tissue and to induce bleeding. The bleeding leads to clot formation and release of growth factors, thus converting a chronic, non-healing injury into an acute injury with increased healing potential (Finnoff *et al.* 2011).

This technique is usually carried out under local anaesthetic and is usually a day operation. A simple technique to replicate this is to use a wide-gauge needle (.30) and to lift and thrust the needle along the Achilles tendon both medially and laterally. The needle is inserted at the myotendinous junction where the gastrocnemius blends into the Achilles tendon. After lifting and thrusting, the needles can be left in place and EA can be applied.

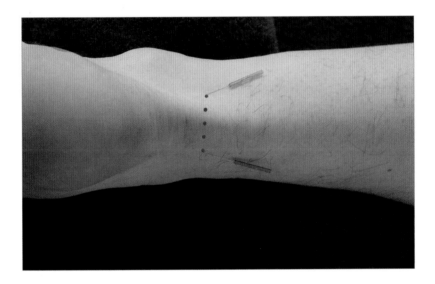

Supraspinatus

The anatomy of the shoulder hinders any direct manual stimulation of the supraspinatus tendon, as it lies deep to the acromial–clavicular joint. The advantage of acupuncture is that it is possible to directly needle into the tendon (Kastner 2014). Calcification of the rotator cuff tendons is common, with around 22 per cent of all rotator cuff pathology having signs of calcification.

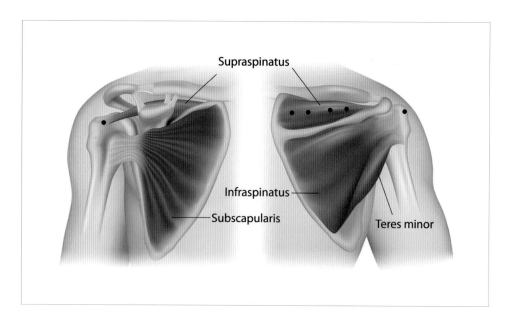

Figure 13.4 Supraspinatus points

Castillo-González *et al.* (2014) considered acupuncture to be a valid alternative as a first-choice treatment of calcific tendinitis of the shoulder. Acupuncture has a number of advantages due to being a simple, cost-effective procedure that does not require hospitalization, it involves no complications when performed in safe hands, rehabilitation treatment is not required and it shows very few side effects without sequelae, significantly reducing the size of the calcification and pain in the majority of patients.

Acupuncture

The following protocol is a suggestion for supraspinatus treatment:

- Large Intestine 16 – deep needling into the supraspinatus tendon at a 35 to 45 degree angle.

- Triple Burner 14 – at the origin of the deltoid muscle, in the depression which lies posterior and inferior to the lateral extremity of the acromion. This can be needled so that the supraspinatus tendon is affected directly.

- Small Intestine 10 – on the shoulder, directly above the posterior end of the axillary fossa, in the depression inferior to the scapular spine.

- The tip of the coracoid process (can be pecked). Caution is needed so as not to penetrate the brachial plexus, as the coracoid process is the site of attachment for several structures. The tip of the coracoid process can be used as a point on the front of the shoulder that can be used for EA when connected to Small Intestine 10.

EA can be used to create a cross-pattern between these four points from LI-16 to TB-14 and SI-10 to the front of the shoulder.

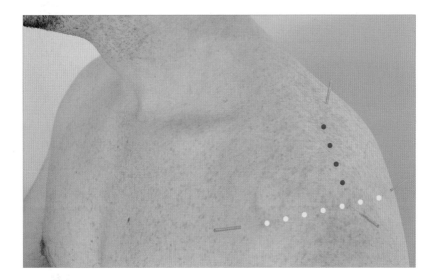

Tennis elbow (lateral epicondylitis)

Lateral epicondylitis, also known as tennis elbow, is significantly more common than medial epicondylitis and has an annual prevalence of 1–2 per cent in the general public. As its common name implies, lateral epicondylitis has a high association with tennis, particularly one-handed backhand strokes. Around 40–50 per cent of recreational tennis players will suffer this condition during their lifetime. The condition, however, is not unique to tennis players. In fact, any sport or occupation that demands repetitive wrist extension can result in this injury (Taylor and Hannafin 2012). Despite the fact that it is often referred to as tennis elbow, this condition occurs more commonly in non-athletes (Marchand *et al.* 2014).

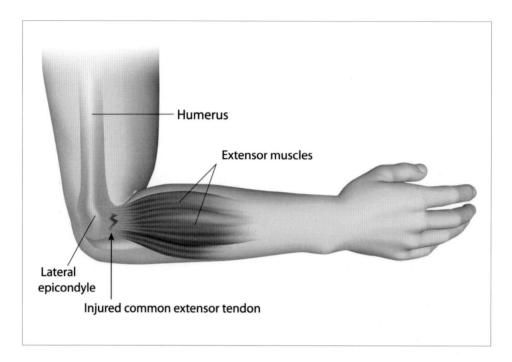

Figure 13.5 Tennis elbow (right arm, lateral side)

As a result of recent evidence, this condition should now be classified as common extensor tendinopathy. Extensor tendinopathy is usually caused by activities that require repetitive use of the muscles that control the wrist, hand and fingers. The problem is felt in the tendons or common extensor origin (CEO) of these muscles, on the outside of the arm. The overuse of these muscles can cause tiny tearing and degeneration or breakdown of the tendon. This series of events then leads to an increased blood vessel growth that relates to an increase in pain rather than healing. This is further complicated by an increase of nerve fibres. These new fibres pick up painful stimuli and this coincides with an increase in pain-producing chemicals to the area. It can become a very painful and debilitating condition.

All of the major extensor muscles of the elbow have one attachment point – the lateral epicondyle – and all form into one tendon, the common extensor tendon. The extensor carpi radialis brevis (ECRB) is the most commonly affected tendon, although other tendons in the extensor bundle can be affected. Lateral epicondylitis is clinically defined by pain at the origin of the common extensor tendon on the lateral epicondyle of the humerus, with maximal tenderness usually less than 0.2 inches distal and anterior to the midpoint of the proximal muscular insertions.

Acupuncture

Palpate for tenderness around the epicondyle where the common extensor attaches, and along all of the extensors, supinator and triceps.

Needle the worst one-to-four points (close to Large Intestine 11) around the epicondyle with or without periosteal pecking. Use EA across the joint or along the extensor group for stimulation of a wider area.

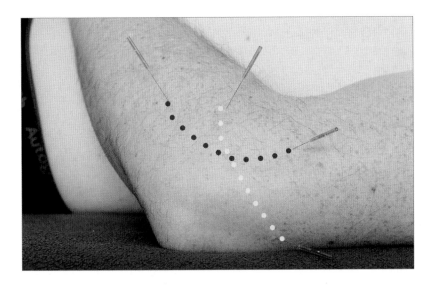

Golfer's elbow (medial epicondylitis)

Medial epicondylitis is known as golfer's elbow, but also occurs often in those who participate in a variety of other sports and occupational activities that create valgus force at the elbow. These are primarily throwing sports. Again, due to histopathology, it should be referred to as common flexor tendon tendinopathy. Tendinopathy results when long-term overuse of the tendons continues, resulting in inadequate repair mechanisms. The pathogenesis of medial epicondylitis parallels that of lateral epicondylitis, beginning with repetitive microtrauma to the wrist flexors originating at their insertion on the medial epicondyle. The diagnosis is made based on history, tenderness at the epicondyle on palpation, and resisted isometric flexion of the wrist provoking symptoms, as well as differential diagnosis.

The musculotendinous structures around the medial epicondyle include multiple muscles. From proximal to distal, these are the pronator teres, the flexor carpi radialis, the palmaris longus, the flexor digitorum superficialis and the flexor carpi ulnaris (Jobe and Ciccotti 1994). The muscles most commonly involved include the pronator teres and flexor carpi radialis but can include any of the other flexors, and therefore all flexor muscles should be palpated.

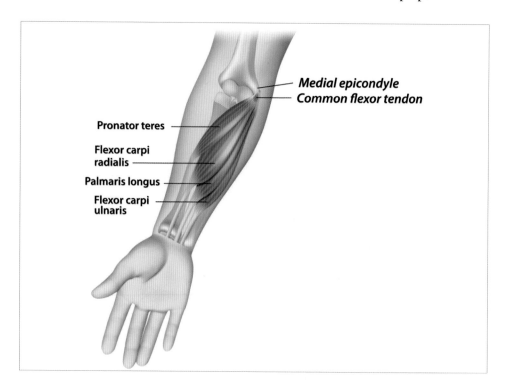

Figure 13.6 Golfer's elbow

Acupuncture

Needling around the medial epicondyle must be done with caution due to the close proximity of the ulnar nerve. Search for trigger points in all of the flexors, as this may cause or contribute to ulnar compressive neuropathy and degrade the tendon due to excessive force placed on the tendon. The technique is the same as for tennis elbow. Needle the worst one-to-four points around the epicondyle with or without periosteal pecking. Use EA across the joint or along the flexor group for stimulation of a wider area.

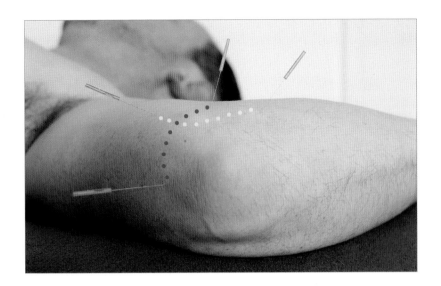

High hamstring tendinopathy

High hamstring tendinopathy (HHT) is an overuse injury that occurs most commonly in distance runners. Symptoms include deep gluteal region pain that is aggravated by running or brisk walking. In severe cases, symptoms may also be aggravated by sitting on hard surfaces. Limited information is available on the diagnosis and treatment of HHTs, but histologic studies have shown dense fibrosis at the hamstring attachment to the ischial tuberosity. Running is thought to place the hamstrings at risk for injury because of the large amount of time that the muscle group spends under maximal stretch and because of repetitive eccentric loading into this position (McCormack 2012). Again, conservative treatment is based on eccentric training to strengthen the hamstrings, but evidence is lacking, and the benefits have not been thoroughly studied.

Fredericson *et al.* (2005) describe the anatomy of the hamstrings as consisting of three muscles: the semitendinosus, the semimembranosus and the biceps femoris (long and short heads). All three muscles, except for the short head of the biceps femoris, originate from the ischial tuberosity as an incompletely separated tendinous mass. The separate muscles become distinguishable 2–4 inches from the tuberosity. All patients should be assessed for pain, thickening and tightness around the ischial tuberosity. This fibrosis around the ischial tuberosity can cause entrapment of the sciatic nerve.

Differential diagnosis is important, and the practitioner should screen for lumbosacral dysfunction, hamstring flexibility, piriformis syndrome, sacroiliac joint (SIJ) dysfunction and other conditions.

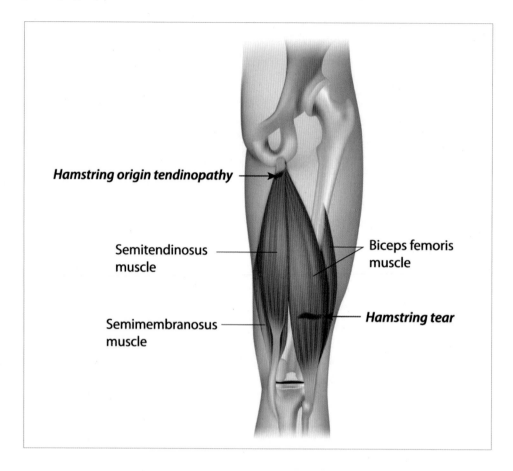

Figure 13.7 Hamstring injury (right leg, dorsal view)

Acupuncture

Palpate for the ischial tuberosity. This can be needled directly, and periosteal pecking can be applied. The needle can be left in or withdrawn. A cross-pattern technique can then be applied with four needles. Each needle is roughly 0.5–1 inch from the ischial tuberosity and placed superior, inferior, medial and lateral to the ischial tuberosity. The needles can be angled towards the tuberosity into the fibrous mass of the tendon. EA can then be applied from superior to inferior and medial to lateral. Palpate for trigger points in the hamstrings, gluteus and piriformis, and needle if appropriate. Segmental points can be added at the levels of L-4/L-5, and EA can be applied.

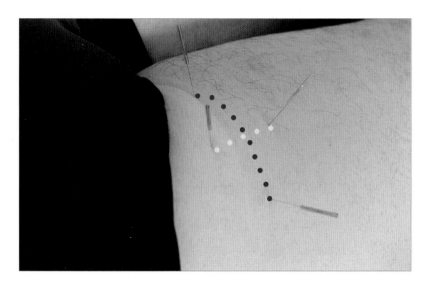

Patellar tendinopathy

Chronic patellar tendon conditions, also known as patellar tendinosis or 'jumper's knee', are numerous in elite athletes who run and jump. The posterior proximal patellar tendon is subjected to greater tensile tendinous forces as compared with the anterior region, especially with jumping activities (Rutland *et al.* 2010).

The patellar tendon, the extension of the common tendon of insertion of the quadriceps femoris muscle, extends from the inferior pole of the patella to the tibial tuberosity (Khan *et al.* 1998). The microtrauma to the posterior proximal patellar tendon or 'overuse' injury develops from repetitive mechanical loading of the tendon, typically through excessive jumping and landing activity. As with all tendons, any major changes in frequency and/ or intensity of training may also lead to overuse and overload of the tendon (Rutland *et al.* 2010). In addition, other factors may have an impact, such as quick acceleration and deceleration, stopping and sudden rotation, causing compressive and shear forces on the tendon.

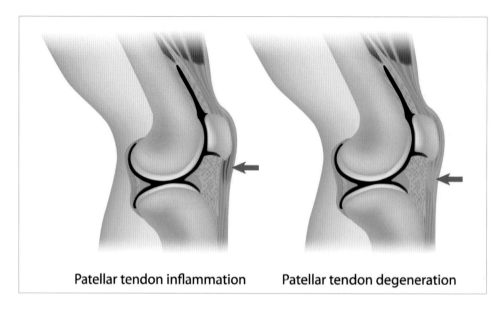

Patellar tendon inflammation   Patellar tendon degeneration

Figure 13.8 Knee injury (jumper's knee)

The blood supply has been postulated to contribute to patellar tendinopathy; however, at rest it has a well-vascularized blood supply which may suddenly be reduced during physical activity. The patellar tendon receives its blood supply through the anastomotic ring, which lies in the thin layers of loose connective tissue covering the dense fibrous expansion of the rectus femoris (Khan *et al.* 1998). Needling into this area will help blood flow into the tendon.

Physical examination should look for pain at the tendon insertion, and any thickness should be noted. Additional functional tests such as single leg squats should be performed, and jumping tests should be used as provocation tests.

Treatment for patellar tendinopathy often includes stretching of lower limb muscles, deep friction massage across the patellar tendon and eccentric quadriceps exercises. Acupuncture can be utilized as part of this conservative programme.

Acupuncture

Needle the following points:

- eyes of the knee

- Stomach 36

- Spleen 9.

Retain for between 20 and 30 minutes. EA can be applied to create a cross-pattern diagonally across the patella tendon.

Additional points to needle to add to the suggested protocol are Stomach 34 and Spleen 10.

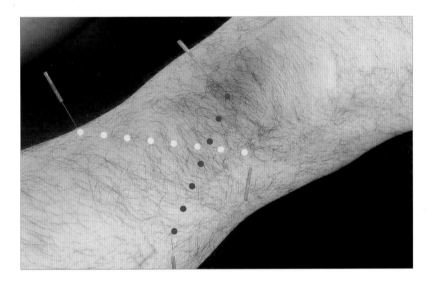

De Quervain's

De Quervain's stenosing tenosynovitis is a disorder that is characterized by wrist pain and tenderness at the radial styloid. It is caused by impaired gliding of the tendons of the abductor pollicis longus (APL) and extensor pollicis brevis (EPB) muscles. These musculotendinous units control the position and orientation, force application and joint stability of the thumb. The impaired gliding is believed to be as a result of thickening of the extensor retinaculum at the first dorsal (extensor) compartment of the wrist, with subsequent narrowing at the fibro-osseous canal (Papa 2012).

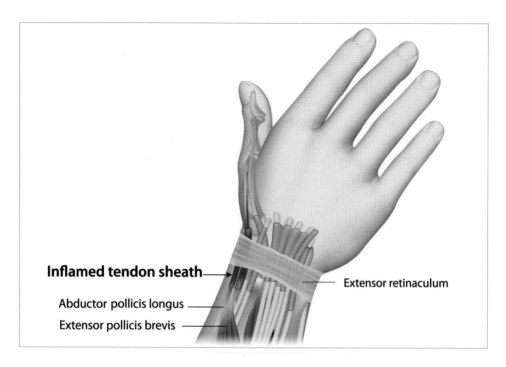

Inflamed tendon sheath

Abductor pollicis longus

Extensor pollicis brevis

Extensor retinaculum

Figure 13.9 De Quervain's Syndrome

Acupuncture

Thread needle along the tendons of the thumb. Thread needle lateral to the extensor pollicis longus, then needle lateral to the abductor pollicis longus. Needle two other points: a trigger point near the styloid process, and another near or on Large Intestine 6. EA can be applied to create a cross-pattern diagonally that runs across the tendon.

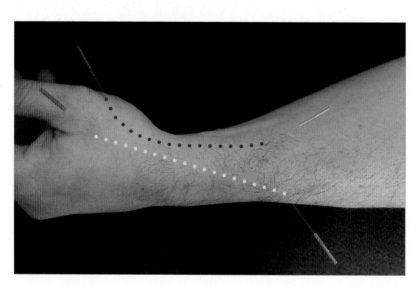

Plantar fasciitis

The plantar fascia is a band of fibrous tissue that originates from the medial tubercle of the calcaneus and stretches to the proximal phalanx of each toe. It is the main stabilizer of the medial arch of the foot against ground reactive forces, and is instrumental in reconfiguring the foot into a rigid platform before toe-off. Sudden changes in the intensity, duration and frequency of loading the lower limb may overload the supporting structures of the lower extremity, eventually leading to injury (Dubin 2007).

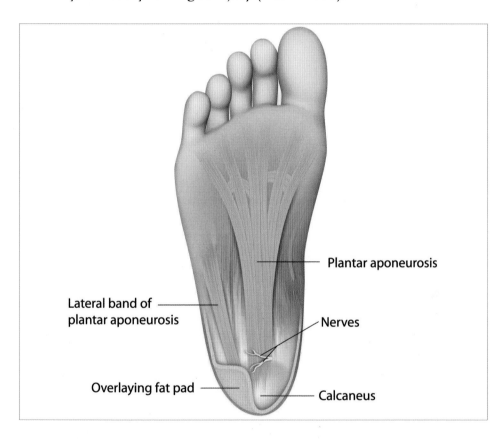

Figure 13.10 Plantar fascia

Plantar fasciitis is thought to be caused by biomechanical overuse from prolonged standing or running, thus creating microtears at the calcaneal enthesis. Some experts have deemed this condition 'plantar fasciosis', implying that its aetiology is a more chronic degenerative process versus acute inflammation (Goff and Crawford 2011). The plantar fascia is a common source of heel pain.

Various risk factors can be contributory, including excessive foot pronation, excessive loading of lower limb (running, walking, prolonged standing, etc.), high arches, obesity and overly tight calf muscles.

Diagnosis is usually based on clinical signs taken in conjunction with a complete case history. The clinical signs include: plantar heel pain when weight-bearing after a period of non-weight-bearing; pain that eases with initial activity; and pain that is usually worse in the morning.

Conservative treatment for plantar fasciitis often includes restoring range of motion and strength in lower limb muscles, correcting training errors and limiting biomechanical deviations (orthotics/insoles) and manual therapy into the plantar fascia.

Acupuncture

For heel pain, a four-needle cross-pattern technique can be used. Each needle is inserted into the tissue of the heel – two on the lateral side and two on the medial side. Needle insertion can be painful, so press hard on the guide tube and insert the needle quickly to cause minimum discomfort. EA can then be applied to run diagonally across the heel.

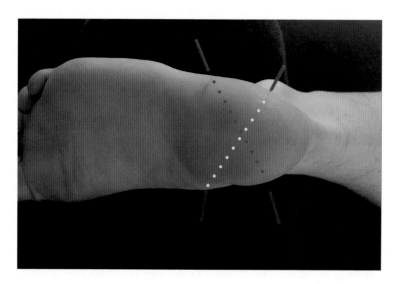

For pain in the plantar fascia, needle into the band itself, usually on the medial side. Two to four needles can be used, depending on patient tolerance. EA can be applied to the superior and inferior needles so that the current runs through the band of tissue.

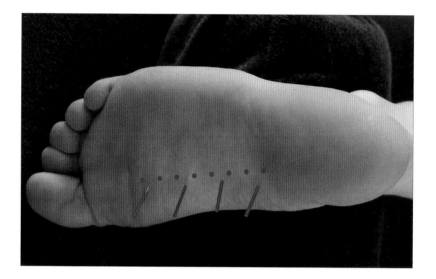

If shortened calf muscles are part of the clinical picture, then needling these muscles can be included in the treatment plan (e.g. Bladder 55/56/57/58).

Tibialis posterior syndrome

Kirby (2000, p.2) describes the anatomy of the tibialis tendon as:

> originating from the posterior aspects of the tibia, fibula, and interosseous membrane as the deepest muscle in the deep posterior compartment of the leg. The posterior tendon passes posterior to the medial malleolus within the confines of the flexor retinaculum, just slightly posterior to the ankle joint axis. As the tendon continues inferior to the medial malleolus, it passes medial and plantar to the subtalar joint axis and plantar to the oblique midtarsal joint axis. Just posterior to the navicular tuberosity, the tendon divides into three components: anterior, middle, and posterior. The anterior component is the largest of the tendon components, sending insertions to the navicular tuberosity and plantar aspect of the first cuneiform. The middle component inserts deeply in the plantar arch of the foot onto the second and third cuneiforms, the cuboid, and onto the bases of the second through fifth metatarsals (the fifth metatarsal insertion is sometimes absent). The posterior component branches laterally and posteriorly and inserts onto the anterior aspect of the sustentaculum tali.

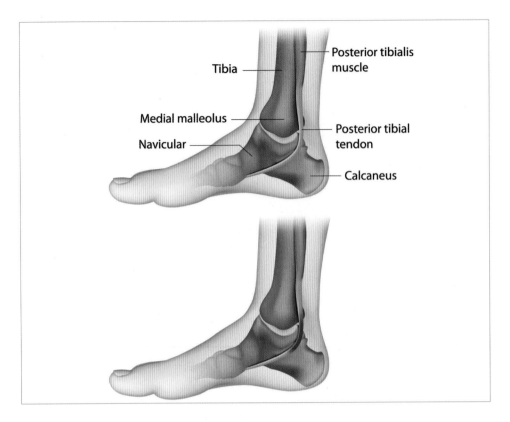

Figure 13.11 Posterior tibial tendon dysfunction

The tibialis posterior tendon is the primary dynamic stabilizer of the medial longitudinal arch. Its contraction results in inversion and plantar flexion of the foot and serves to elevate the medial longitudinal arch, which locks the mid-tarsal bones, making the hind foot and midfoot rigid (Kohls-Gatzoulis *et al.* 2004).

It has been proposed that the tibialis posterior tendon becomes fibrotic through a process of repeated microtrauma. In addition, a poor blood supply to the tendon has been identified as it courses posterior to the medial malleolus, leaving it susceptible to regeneration in that area. A growing body of research proposes that abnormal forces arise from even mild flatfootedness, resulting in lifelong greater mechanical demands on the tibialis posterior than in a normal foot. Most people who develop the condition already have flat feet (Kohls-Gatzoulis *et al.* 2004). With overuse or continuous loading, a change occurs where the arch begins to flatten more than before, with pain and swelling developing on the inside of the ankle. Inadequate support from footwear may occasionally be a contributing factor. Other factors include trauma or injury to the lower limb, and occasionally this condition may be due to fracture, sprain or a direct blow to the tendon. The risk of developing posterior tibial tendon dysfunction increases with age, and research has suggested that middle-aged women are more commonly affected.

Typically, tibialis posterior tendinopathy is classified into four stages:

- *Stage 1.* Medial malleolus pain and swelling along the tendon. The patient is able to stand on tiptoe on one leg and is usually treated with insoles and manual therapy. In the later stages the patient will have developed an acquired flatfoot deformity.

- *Stage 2.* The patient will have more pain and swelling than in Stage 1, with increased flattening of the foot and decreased power in the tendon. Tendon reconstruction is necessary if conservative treatment fails.

- *Stage 3.* A degree of deformity at the subtalar joint is found on X-ray. It may be treated with the use of orthoses. A fusion of the hind foot may be necessary.

- *Stage 4.* Accompanying ankle deformity. Surgery to the ankle may be necessary.

In Stage 1 of tibialis posterior dysfunction, the signs are of swelling and tenderness behind and below the medial malleolus (along the course of the tendon), and some weakness or pain with inversion of the foot. The patient may have some difficulty rising on one heel only, or weakness after multiple heel rises.

When palpating along the tibialis posterior tendon, look for swelling, signs of deformity and pain on palpation, all of which are signs of dysfunction. Other tests include visual inspection of the foot (looking for heel alignment and flat foot) and testing the tendon for power (with posterior tibial dysfunction, the posterior tibial muscle contraction is unable to generate adequate tensile forces in the posterior tibial tendon). A functional test is to ask the patient to perform ten heel raises (patients with tibialis posterior dysfunction will not be able to do this).

Acupuncture

Acupuncture may be of use in tendon regeneration and pain reduction primarily in Stages 1 and 2 alongside conservative management. In Stages 3 and 4 its use is mainly for pain management. Use the suggested points below to create a cross-pattern and to increase blood flow to the tendon:

- Kidney 2 to Kidney 7

- Spleen 4 to Spleen 6.

EA can be applied to stimulate a greater area across the tendon from Kidney 2 to Kidney 7 and from Spleen 4 to Spleen 6. Check for trigger points in the peroneals and lateral leg muscles.

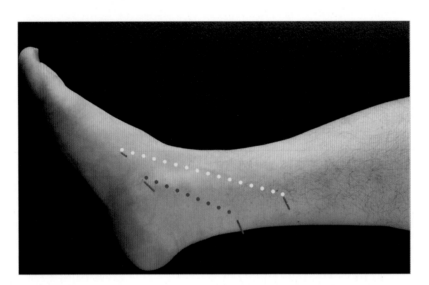

References

Abate, M. (2014) 'How obesity modifies tendons (implications for athletic activities).' *Muscles, Ligaments and Tendons Journal 4*, 3, 298–302.

Alfredson, H., and Cook, J. (2007) 'A treatment algorithm for managing Achilles tendinopathy: new treatment options.' *Br. J. Sports Med. 41*, 211–216.

Arnoczky, S.P., Lavagnino, M., and Egerbacher, M. (2007) 'The mechanobiological aetiopathogenesis of tendinopathy: is it the over-stimulation or the under-stimulation of tendon cells?' *International Journal of Experimental Pathology 88*, 4, 217–226.

BMJ (2012) 'Management of chronic Achilles tendinopathy.' *Drug and Therapeutics Bulletin 50*, 93–96.

Borchers, J., Krey, D., and McCamey, K. (2015) 'Tendon needling for treatment of tendinopathy: a systematic review.' *The Physician and Sportsmedicine 43*, 1, 80–86.

Castillo-González, F., Ramos-Álvarez, J., Rodríguez-Fabián, G., González-Pérez, J., and Calderón-Montero, J. (2014) 'Treatment of the calcific tendinopathy of the rotator cuff by ultrasound-guided percutaneous needle lavage: two years prospective study.' *Muscles, Ligaments and Tendons Journal 4*, 2, 220–225.

Charvet, B., Ruggiero, F., and Le Guellec, D. (2012) 'The development of the myotendinous junction: a review.' *Muscles, Ligaments and Tendons Journal 2*, 2, 53–63.

Cook, J., Khan, M., and Purdam, C. (2002) 'Achilles tendinopathy.' *Manual Therapy 7*, 3, 121–130.

De Almeida, M.D.S., De Freitas, K.M., and De Oliveira, L.P. (2015) 'Acupuncture increases the diameter and reorganisation of collagen fibrils during rat tendon healing.' *Acupunct. Med. 33*, 51–57.

De Almeida, M.D.S., Guerra, F.D.R., De Oliveira, L.P., Vieira, C.P., and Pimentel, E.R.A. (2014) 'Hypothesis for the anti-inflammatory and mechanotransduction molecular mechanisms underlying acupuncture tendon healing.' *Acupunct. Med. 32*, 2, 178–182.

Dubin, J. (2007) 'Evidence based treatment for plantar fasciitis.' *Sports Therapy.* Available at http://dubinchiro.com/plantar.pdf, accessed on 27 July 2015.

Fahlström, M., Jonsson, P., Lorentzon, R., and Alfredson, H. (2003) 'Chronic Achilles tendon pain treated with eccentric calf-muscle training.' *Knee Surg. Sports Traumatol. Arthrosc. 1*, 5, 327.

Finnoff, J.T., Fowler, S.P., Lai, J.K., *et al.* (2011) 'Treatment of chronic tendinopathy with ultrasound-guided needle tenotomy and platelet-rich plasma injection.' *American Academy of Physical Medicine and Rehabilitation (AAPM&R) 3*, 10, 900–911.

Fredericson, M., Moore, W., Guillet, M., and Beaulieu, C. (2005) 'High hamstring tendinopathy in runners: meeting the challenges of diagnosis, treatment, and rehabilitation.' *Phys. Sportsmed. 33*, 5, 32–43.

Goff, J.G., and Crawford, R. (2011) 'Diagnosis and treatment of plantar fasciitis.' *American Family Physician 84*, 6, 676–682.

Hansson, Y., Carlsson, C., and Olsson, E. (2008) 'Intramuscular and periosteal acupuncture in patients suffering from chronic musculoskeletal pain – a controlled trial.' *Acupunct. Med. 26*, 4, 214–223.

Inoue, M., Nakajima, M., Oi, Y., Hojo, T., Itoi, M., and Kitakoji, H. (2015) 'The effect of electroacupuncture on tendon repair in a rat Achilles tendon rupture model.' *Acupunct. Med. 33*, 58–64.

Jobe, F., and Ciccotti, M. (1994) 'Lateral and medial epicondylitis of the elbow.' *Journal of the American Academy of Orthopaedic Surgeons 2*, 1, 1–8.

Kastner, M. (2014) 'The treatment of tendon pain with traditional Chinese medicine.' *Journal of Chinese Medicine 106*, 12–20.

Khan, K. (2003) 'The painful nonruptured tendon: clinical aspects.' *Clin. Sports Med. 22*, 711–725.

Khan, K.M., Maffulli, N., Coleman, B.D., Cook, J.L., and Taunton, J.E. (1998) 'Patellar tendinopathy: some aspects of basic science and clinical management.' *British Journal of Sports Medicine 32*, 4, 346–355.

Kirby, K.A. (2000) *Conservative Treatment of Posterior Tibial Dysfunction.* Online. Available at http://podiatrym.com/cme/September200Kirby.pdf, accessed on 27 July 2015.

Kishmishian, B., Selfe, J., and Richards, J. (2012) 'A historical review of acupuncture to the Achilles tendon and the development of a standardized protocol for its use.' *Journal of the Acupuncture Association of Chartered Physiotherapists*, Spring 2012, *69–78*. Available at www.researchgate.net/publication/232946047_A_historical_review_of_acupuncture_to_the_Achilles_tendon_and_the_development_of_a_standardized_protocol_for_its_use, accessed on 27 July 2015.

Kohls-Gatzoulis, J., Angel, J.C., Singh, D., Haddad, F., Livingstone, J., and Berry, G. (2004) 'Tibialis posterior dysfunction: a common and treatable cause of adult acquired flatfoot.' *British Medical Journal 329*, 7478, 1328–1333.

Kubo, K., Yajima, H., Takayama, M., Ikebukuro, T., Mizoguchi, H., and Takakura, N. (2010) 'Effects of acupuncture and heating on blood volume and oxygen saturation of human Achilles tendon in-vivo.' *Eur. J. Appl. Physiol. 109*, 545–550.

Leadbetter, W.B. (1992) 'Cell-matrix response in tendon injury.' *Clin. Sports Med. 11*, 3, 533–578.

Mann, F. (2000) *Reinventing Acupuncture: A New Concept of Ancient Medicine* (second edition). Oxford: Butterworth-Heinemann.

Marchand, A.-A., O'Shaughnessy, J., and Descarreaux, M. (2014) 'Humeral lateral epicondylitis complicated by hydroxyapatite dihydrite deposition disease: a case report.' *Journal of Chiropractic Medicine 13*, 1, 67–74.

McCormack, J. (2012) 'The management of bilateral high hamstring tendinopathy with ASTYMH treatment and eccentric exercise: a case report.' *Journal of Manual and Manipulative Therapy 20*, 3, 142–146.

McCreesh, K., and Lewis, J. (2013) 'Continuum model of tendon pathology – where are we now?' *International Journal of Experimental Pathology 94*, 242–247.

Nantel, J., Mathieu, M.-E., and Prince, F. (2011) 'Physical activity and obesity: biomechanical and physiological key concepts.' *Journal of Obesity 2011*, 650230.

Neal, B., and Longbottom, J. (2012) 'Is there a role for acupuncture in the treatment of tendinopathy?' *Acupuncture in Medicine 30*, 4, 346–349.

Papa, J. (2012) 'Conservative management of De Quervain's stenosing tenosynovitis: a case report.' *J. Can. Chiropr. Assoc. 56*, 2, 112–120.

Rees, J.D., Stride, M., and Scott, A. (2013) 'Tendons – time to revisit inflammation.' *Br. J. Sports Med.* Online. Available at http://bjsm.bmj.com/content/early/2013/03/08/bjsports-2012-091957.full, accessed on 27 July 2015.

Rutland, M., O'Connell, D., Brismée, J.-M., Sizer, P., Apte, G., and O'Connell, J. (2010) 'Evidence-supported rehabilitation of patellar tendinopathy.' *North American Journal of Sports Physical Therapy 5*, 3, 166–178.

Selvanetti, A., Cipolla, M., and Puddu, G. (1997) 'Overuse tendon injuries: basic science and classification.' *Operative Techniques in Sports Medicine 5*, 3, 110–117.

Sharma, P., and Maffulli, N. (2005) 'Tendon injury and tendinopathy: healing and repair.' *J. Bone Joint Surg. Am. 87*, 187–202.

Speed, C. (2015) 'Acupuncture's role in tendinopathy: new possibilities.' *Acupuncture in Medicine 33*, 1, 7–8.

Taylor, S.A., and Hannafin, J.A. (2012) 'Evaluation and management of elbow tendinopathy.' *Sports Health 4*, 5, 384–393.

Xu, Y., and Murrell, G.A.C. (2008) 'The basic science of tendinopathy.' *Clinical Orthopaedics and Related Research 466*, 7, 1528–1538.

Zhao, Z.-Q. (2008) 'Neural mechanism underlying acupuncture analgesia.' *Progress in Neurobiology 85*, 355–375.

Subject Index

Author Index